I0145942

FLOWER POWER

Essences That Heal

Second Edition

SENECA SCHURBON

Copyright © 2013 and
Second edition copyright © 2020 by Seneca Schurbon

All rights reserved. This book is protected by the copyright laws of the United States of America. No portion of this book may be stored electronically, transmitted, copied, reproduced, or reprinted for commercial gain or profit without prior written permission from Seneca Schurbon. Permission requests may be emailed to seneca@freedom-flowers.com. Only the use of short quotations for reviews or as reference material in other works is allowed without written permission.

All Scripture quotations, unless otherwise indicated, are taken from the New International Version®, NIV®. Copyright ©1973, 1978, 1984, 2011 by Biblica, Inc.™ Used by permission of Zondervan. All rights reserved worldwide. www.zondervan.com The "NIV" and "New International Version" are trademarks registered in the United States Patent and Trademark Office by Biblica, Inc.™

Scripture taken from the New King James Version® is marked as (NKJV). Copyright © 1982 by Thomas Nelson. Used by permission. All rights reserved.

Scripture taken from the King James Version are marked as (KJV). Public domain.

ISBN 978-1-7333795-1-9

The information contained in "*Flower Power: Essences That Heal*" is not meant to take the place of professional, medical, or psychotherapeutic care. This book is a reference work not intended to treat, diagnose, or prescribe medical conditions or illness. Results are not guaranteed and may vary with use.

DEDICATION

To my husband Mike and dog Zoe, without whom there
would be no business and no book!

CONTENTS

Dedication. 3

Introduction 1

What Are Flower Essences? 5

Eden in Our Hearts. 11

How Flowers Can Change Your Life 19

Flower Essences and Physical Healing 27

Trauma 39

How to Choose and Use Your Essences 45

Helping Animals with Flower Essences 59

Q & A. 69

Freedom Flowers A–Z .75

Bouquet Blends 119

Thank You! 125

About the Author 129

Other Books by the Author 131

INTRODUCTION

THIS LITTLE BOOK will change the way you handle bad moods, emotional woundings, negative thought processes, and coping methods that cause more problems than they solve. You won't have to try to "think positive" or attempt to control and redirect your thoughts; you'll just effortlessly operate on a plane above those issues.

You won't have to do a bunch of tapping or repeat affirmations over and over, hoping it works. The most effort you'll have to make is to remember to put four virtually tasteless drops into your drink and take a sip now and then.

Flower essences can either offer deep healing or provide fine-tuning, depending on your personal needs. People use them for everything from addressing old childhood woundings to increasing their productivity. I made myself a book-writing blend to help me organize this information, communicate it clearly, and believe in my own voice. Did it work? You'll have to tell me!

I started making flower essences intuitively when I was little, in no way fathoming the magnitude of what I was doing. I didn't grow up in a family that was particularly focused on alternative medicine. Back then, I was just having fun with flowers. I had the basic technique down but no quality control standards. I bottled my flower essences in empty film canisters and sold them for seventy-five cents each. Who knew I was onto something big here?

These days, those original essences—Harebell, Sweet Pea, and Daisies—are still part of my repertoire. Quality control these days is stringent, and most of the flowers come from where I live: on the edge of the Selway Bitterroot Wilderness in Idaho.

If you like side benefits instead of side effects and simple and natural methodology with a safety record that can't be beat, essences are perfect for you. This will be a quick but thorough introduction for the newbie that will give you the confidence to work with essences either on your own or with a practitioner. The seasoned essence user will turn to the A-Z essence section again and again as a reference guide.

Don't waste any more time struggling with negative emotions and the effects they have on your relationships, your health, your career, and the decisions you make in every area of life. This book is a quick read so that you can start your healing process. You have my permission to skip to the back and start picking flowers.

My goal is for the world to realize and experience the gentleness, power, depth, and tremendous versatility of flower healing. Indeed, our Creator uses the "foolish things of the world to confound the wise" (1 Corinthians 1:27 KJV).

WHAT ARE FLOWER ESSENCES?

I N A NUTSHELL, flower essences are the energetic frequency of a flower that has been imprinted onto water and preserved. Flower essences capitalize on flowers' vibrational frequencies to alter negative emotional patterns. Flower essences can reverse trauma, anxiety, depression, and patterns of negative thinking.

We have used plants for millennia to heal. Since we're dealing with *frequencies* rather than with *biochemical processes*, flower essences capture the most robust expression of this energy vibration. The flowering part of any plant is its reproductive apparatus, so each plant spends its energy on the flower to complete its life cycle. In the essence-making process, we transfer the *flower frequency* to water because water is a perfect carrier and recorder for transferring energy to the body. Water transports the flowers' frequencies into the body. Although flower essences don't directly affect the body, they correct the emotional components that contribute to disease, so many people and pets enjoy emotional and physical relief.

Please don't confuse flower essences with the essential oils used in aromatherapy. Essential oils are made from the aromatic parts of plants, not necessarily the flowers. Flower essences have no scent, and you typically ingest them; we usually apply essential oils to the skin or diffuse them. Oils have physical components that heal while flower essences are purely energetic. Since they operate on an energetic level rather than a physical one, you won't have drug interactions, allergic reactions, or contraindications.

To understand how flower essences can affect your emotional well-being, you'll need to understand how humans perceive frequencies. *Everything in existence emanates a unique, trademark frequency.* Your body picks up energetic frequencies in various ways: seeing, hearing, tasting, feeling and smelling are the most common of these. This is why you're often noticeably affected by sounds, colors, lights, and scents.

Every emotion you experience has a unique frequency. Negative emotions— anger and fear—vibrate at lower-frequency ranges; positive emotions— love and joy— vibrate at higher ranges. Unconditional love resonates at the highest frequency. *To change your emotional state, you have to change your frequency.* Raising a fear-level frequency causes you to move away from fear and toward peace, joy, and love. In the realm of physics, this is how perfect love casts out all fear. (See 1 John 4:18.)

If you take two tuning forks in two different pitches and twang them simultaneously, the vibration of each will express two distinct pitches—but only at first. As the two forks continue to vibrate, the one with the lower power gradually adopts the frequency of the one with the higher power. They begin to sound alike.

This is very similar to what happens when you take an appropriate flower essence: suddenly you have more than one pitch happening at the same time. So for example, if an old thought pattern that tells you "I can't forgive, I'm too angry" is suddenly paired with "I can love you anyway," you may perceive the newest frequency as a choice or a new idea. You then begin to entertain the notion that there *is* another way to react to your circumstances. As you continue to infuse the higher frequency, your choice becomes clearer, and the old patterns (the lower-resonating frequencies) change. The higher frequency causes the old vibration to yield to something that *feels* better (is less stressful or anxiety-provoking) than what you've been experiencing.

Again, each flower resonates at its trademark specific frequency. This frequency is then transferred to water—the perfect recorder, conductor, and carrier. When you transfer a few drops of a flower essence to a glass of water, your entire glass is encoded with that specific frequency, and every time you take a sip or apply it topically, your body, which is approximately 70 percent water, becomes infused with a specific frequency that can build you up in ways that hundreds of dollars invested in self-help books can't.

Flower essences are subtle, so most people don't immediately recognize how significantly they're shifting and releasing old patterns that keep them stuck and stymied. Your own awareness of transformation will depend on your present degree of self-awareness.

The first time you take an essence, you might struggle to identify what's happening. (This is not always the case.) You simply don't know what to expect. But some new users are immediately and profoundly affected. Quite often, the changes reveal themselves during dreams. For this reason, dream interpretation and flower essence therapy are particularly complimentary. Dreams, positive declarations, prayer and other modalities can accelerate the process.

Flower essences aren't gatecrashers. They don't override personality; they simply help restore who you really are. As you are delivered from heavier, lower-vibration frequencies, you should begin to experience new joy and increased empowerment. You're likely to become increasingly amenable to new experiences, relationships, and opportunities. You should attract fewer problems and be better able to avoid traps that would have easily ensnared you before. Others may even begin to treat you better as your attitude toward yourself improves and begins to flourish. Your decision-making process will likely improve, too, because negative emotions (e.g., fear, self-doubt, and second-guessing) won't cloud your thoughts. But please don't expect a surreal, drug-like feel with flower essences. It's just not going to happen.

And although the application or ingestion of flower essences takes effect immediately, you'll probably need to take them for three weeks to a month to recognize real change. It takes three weeks to learn a new habit, and this is what will be happening. You'll be reversing recalcitrant, knee-jerk ways of reacting to negative circumstances and replacing these with positive responses. By the time you break this pernicious cycle, what used to trigger you will carry less emotional impact. You'll be able to respond as opposed to instinctively reacting in the way a wounded animal does.

So by now, you may be asking, Why flowers? Why not counseling or therapy? Do you really want (or need) to dredge up your polluted past again, reopening the wound? Probably not. If you haven't been helped significantly by now, do you really want to continue with the same old methodology, only to repeat the same old lackluster results?

Healing is so much more than learning to tolerate your problems or to focus on something positive when problems arise or learning to see your problems in a different light. While beneficial, all of these are a far cry from complete healing. Even when you try to deal with the pain in more constructive ways, the pain persists. Although medication to balance brain chemicals is sometimes necessary, it isn't true healing because chemical imbalances are symptoms *not sources* of problems.

For example, Alcoholics Anonymous is about learning to manage a problem. By daily confessing that you are an alcoholic, you agree to own this issue for life. Management of a condition is not freedom. And you want to be free! We all do.

I *am* in favor of prayer, especially via inner healing ministries that go after root causes. But sadly, I've seen a lot of partial breakthroughs, no breakthroughs, or healing that doesn't stick. In some cases, a person is accused of having insufficient faith to be healed or told they won't accept the finished work or told they aren't standing on Scripture. This adds insult to injury instead of considering the likelihood that they simply have never addressed the root cause.

In the gardening world, we all know the difference between breaking off a weed at the soil level versus pulling it out by the roots. If you break it off, everything looks good on the surface for a while, but eventually, the weed comes back. (Fortunately, in the world of flower essences, weeds are some of the most tenacious healers.)

I am not tearing down other healing methods (I use them myself), and I'm not saying to stop what you're doing, but please do consider adding flower essences to the mix. Hit your situation with everything in your arsenal! You're in charge of your recovery process, so you need to decide what's right for you. I ultimately want you to settle on a strategy of never settling for less than going after the roots, no matter which healing modalities you choose.

EDEN IN OUR HEARTS

BELIEVE A PRECEDENT was set and revealed early in the Genesis story—a precedent that I honor each time I create essences. In fact, I see a direct correlation between the creation story and what I believe was God's original intent in creating the garden of Eden.

To be transparent here, I'm not a religious person. *My view of organized religion is that it has fostered evil and ill will for millennia now and, as a sad result, has failed humankind miserably.* That said, I do believe in the God of the Bible. I also believe that we've glossed over a good many keys to healing as well as how injury happens in the first place. Keys contained in the book of Genesis and in other ancient texts essentially relate the same story.

"In the beginning God created the heavens and the earth. Now the earth was formless and empty, darkness was over the surface of the deep, and the Spirit of God was hovering over the waters" (Genesis 1:1–2).

English doesn't do the creation story justice. It's impossible to translate Hebrew to English without losing essential details. Each word has several meanings; even the characters that make up the words possess multiple levels of depth. What I want to point out here is that the word "hover" means to flutter, shake, or vibrate.[1] So the Spirit of God was vibrating over the waters, *infusing them* with divine frequency—fine-tuning the planet we call home to the vibration and sound of its Creator.

Some Bible scholars believe a lot more happened between the two sentences you read above. This may explain why so little science appears to align with typical creationist beliefs. It may also explain why, on the opening page of the original Hebrew text, the earth appears to have *become* a total mess (*tohuw*, meaning chaotic, nothing, confusion, waste, wilderness, empty, formless, and vain)[2] *after* God created it.

A more accurate translation of the original Hebrew might read this way: "In the beginning God created the heavens and the earth. Now the earth *became* chaotic and empty, darkness was over the surface of the deep, and the Spirit of God was vibrating over the waters." (See Genesis 1:1–2, emphasis added.) We see God covering the earth with water a second time in the story of Noah. The passage doesn't specifically say that the same hovering went on in Noah's time, but we do know the dove was sent out from the ark (Genesis 8:8). That was literal, but was it also symbolic? Other Bible references also compare his voice to the sound of water. Psalm 29:3 specifically says the voice of the Lord is over the water.

As I was saying in the last chapter, water is a perfect carrier and recorder of frequency. In fact, it's the only substance on earth that can transmit its frequency to everything that comes into contact with it. Recent research confirms water's ability to bridge energetic and physical worlds by accumulating and transferring vibrational patterns and information.[3] So it only makes sense that God needed to overwrite the intervening broken pattern that resulted in chaos and darkness in order to restore the planet to his original intent.

Here in essence-making land, I use the same process but add the frequency of flowers. I carefully choose the flowers that I add to water, then I pray over the composition and leave it for the Spirit to hover over. That is, I leave the mixture completely untouched until I *literally* see light and see that the light is good. In this careful, conscientious, prayerful way, the flower essences I create are both natural and supernatural.

As a result, my flower essences resonate with the specific healing energy of the flowers I choose and with the energy of the Spirit of God. There is a flower for every emotional disturbance, and I can get ultra-specific when customizing a batch to address an individual's specific challenges.

Flower essences vibrate at extremely high frequencies, which works wonders whenever low-frequency vibrational distur-bances have taken hold of a person. Whenever you introduce a higher-frequency to a lower frequency, the lower frequency *must* yield to the higher frequency. *Always. Without exception.*

Remember water, that perfect carrier and recorder of frequency? As I previously mentioned, our bodies are approximately 70 percent water. Sometimes, old patterns of chaos and darkness needed to be overwritten with a new frequency—our own personal Genesis.

So let's skip ahead to Eden. I believe God's original intent was to bring the kingdom of heaven to Earth. Throughout the Bible, heaven is referred to as a kingdom. If you managed to stay awake in history class, you know that kingdoms and empires expand their territories in one of two ways: by conquest or colonization.

God chose colonization. Even though Earth had a clear and present enemy, war and conquest weren't part of the game plan. Instead, he did the unexpected: he planted a garden!

Inside the garden, he put people and directed them to go forth and multiply. There was a plan for expansion. Eden reflected heaven's atmosphere, government, and culture. There was no sickness, stress, or heartache; there was no decay or corruption. The garden was paradise—heaven on earth. So God's plan was as obvious as the garden itself: occupy Earth and expand his kingdom outward "on earth as it is in heaven."

Although you can no longer find the original Eden on a map, it has become even more accessible. Jesus was crystal clear when he said that restoring God's kingdom on Earth no longer has anything to do with a physical dwelling place. "The kingdom of God does not come with observation; nor will they say, 'See here!' or 'See there!' For indeed, the kingdom of God is within you" (Luke 17:20–21 NKJV).

But restoring God's indwelling kingdom simply can't happen as long as people are carrying chaos, destruction, and wounding inside their bodies.

So far, I've made a good case for water's role in bringing restoration. What about the flowers? Let's take a closer look at the flower's purpose for existing and its end result.

As I said earlier, a flower is the reproductive part of a plant. Its sole purpose is to be fruitful and multiply.

As symbolized in the Bible, fruit refers to attitudes and actions as well as to the outcome of something. Paul said the *fruit* of the Spirit is love, joy, peace, patience, kindness, goodness, faithfulness, gentleness, and self-control. *Flowers always precede fruit*, so it only makes sense that infusing the higher frequency of flowers in water initiates the process that can lead to an idyllic state of being.

Flower essences also make the truth easier to discern. Truth is essential to attaining peace. Most of the time, negative emotions are the result of believing a lie. A lie in this context is anything that disempowers you, anything that causes you to surrender your potential, and anything that is downright false.

In a nutshell, flower essences subtly reframe circumstances, reshape distorted perceptions, and restore favorable states of mind. No wonder we love them so! The following testimony from a satisfied customer shares the power of flower essences.

> When I connected with you, I was in such a deep place of sadness. I received those amazing flower essences, which brought me a much-needed breakthrough. Sometimes when you get break-through in an area it's a battle, and other times it's just a little hump. In this case, it was a battle! I felt as though something were attacking my marriage, my identity, and any forward motion that God was calling me to. The pain and disapproval connected to the mistakes of my past continually came up. The emotions that were connected to those past events tortured me. I wondered how I could handle the pain of past mistakes. I carried the shame, and because I partnered with it, the torment had free reign in my life and made a home there. Crazy weird, I know. But then I started the flower essences.
>
> When taking the drops, I would wake up, start my morning, and thoughts and emotions of hopelessness would return. I instantly remem-bered to ask myself if I had taken the drops. The answer would be no. When I went back and took the drops, my day was great. I had energy and was happy. When the negative thoughts and lies tried to creep back, I could instantly say no. I had

a new-found ability to take authority over my thoughts and would instantly do so. It was as if God used the Freedom Flower Essences to retrain my emotions to take every thought captive.

At the end of thirty days, I was a little nervous. I wasn't sure if my breakthrough was secure. A few weeks went by with normal activity. I was feeling fine with no tormenting thoughts. I just felt healthy and rested. Suddenly, it was as if a bomb dropped, and I had an overwhelming feeling of needing to give. It was as if God filled me up with so much love and joy that I was going to explode! It was a crazy breakthrough of joy, unspeakable joy like I had never experienced. I now feel more authority, hear God more clearly, and walk with a greater understanding of my call. The Father showed me the root issue of where these emotions stemmed from in a dream. He was teaching me how to separate the lies from the truth, and he used the flower essences to do it. My emotions were keeping me from hearing and receiving the truth and heaven's perspective. I learned that my emotions could be a trap that keeps me from connecting to God. So now, I can recognize the negative emotion or lie that keeps me from my God connection. Thank you for the essence that brought truth to my emotional being! ~ Larina Read

HOW FLOWERS CAN
CHANGE YOUR LIFE

F LOWER ESSENCES CAN transform your physical and emotional health. They can also boost your relationships, financial situation, and career. "How is that possible?" you ask.

Because every bad decision you've ever made or destructive behavior you've engaged in was based on a *lie*. When you line up your emotions and core beliefs about yourself with the truth, you become unstoppable, bound for greatness.

Some wrong beliefs came about when you were hurt as a child. Later on, you tried to make sense of it all by leaning on your own imperfect understanding of what happened and what it all meant. All of us inevitably come to wrong conclusions about ourselves and our situations. This leads to feelings of rejection, low self-esteem, and a sense of almost universal distrust of other people. Most people have enormous gaps between how they feel or how they perceive a situation and what the reality actually is—especially if they've been repeatedly wounded.

The sad thing is, we may even intellectually know better than to feel the way we do, but head knowledge never trumps feelings. Rational thinking can identify and perhaps modify a resulting behavior if our reactions don't kick in first, but it can't fix it. At times, we all know what we should do in a given situation, but we do the opposite because we can't override our feelings. We've all been there!

Improving Relationships

It's no surprise that negative emotions cause people to behave badly even within relationships we cherish. We've all experienced the boil-over effect even though we know better. But we still fall victim to misguided behavior.

Simply controlling your feelings and keeping your mouth shut is not a suitable solution. For one thing, internalized, repressed feelings eventually manifest in physical health challenges, which we'll cover in the next chapter. It takes immense energy to squelch something that wants to come out in an inappropriate way. And good luck with depending on your will power to behave better!

Your feelings will win, hands down. Feelings precede thoughts, and thoughts precede actions—usually quicker than you can get a handle on them.

For instance, I tend to have a smart mouth when I believe I'm not being heard or understood. It isn't that I rationally decide, "This situation will improve if I smart off!" Instead, I feel something passionately, and before I can make a conscious rational decision, my feelings are flying out of my mouth!

Flower essences aren't about bolstering self-control; they're about *eliminating* negative emotions, self-limiting beliefs, and healing the old wounds that cause us to *react* feverishly rather than *respond rationally* and more appropriately.

Water boils at 212 degrees. At 210 degrees, you see nothing but steam. Consider this analogy with regard to your feelings. It takes a lot of heat to get you to boil over! You don't escalate from zero to boiling in an instant. More realistically, you accumulate your experiences and your feelings about them over a period of time.

It's easy to forgive someone you've only known for moments when they foul up in some way, but when loved ones, co-workers, and other ever-present people (those important relationships) mess up, we can live our lives at 210 degrees and reach the boiling point at warp speed. You know it happens. It can happen to me too. It's why I keep flower essences close at hand!

But what if we elected to live at 80 degrees instead of at 210 degrees? We'd be able to deal with others' behaviors in constructive ways instead of boiling over as often as we do.

Every seed produces its own kind. Every action and the words you speak in response to what you're feeling will eventually produce more of that same feeling. You simply cannot be driven by negative emotions if your goal is to produce healthy, positive outcomes.

The more your feelings drive your behaviors, the more you'll find yourself in difficult circumstances. The more you'll feel stressed out and the more susceptible to disease you'll become.

There's a better way.

Flower Essences and Your Destiny

Your limiting beliefs about yourself, your fears, your old traumas, and trapped emotions keep you from embracing life and saying yes to the right opportunities. Staying inside a dysfunctional comfort zone usually seems safer than stepping into your potential and a better destiny. It may seem easier just to keep doing what you've been doing, but is it really? Playing small doesn't serve you, your loved ones, or the world.

The good news is that once you deal with negative emotions, truth becomes your default setting. It will resonate to the core of your being, and the lower, heavier frequencies will yield to your higher, more powerful vibration. You'll begin to feel more like Wonder Woman and Superman than you ever have before.

You have ambitions and dreams. Your present beliefs and feelings play a major role in how well you access what you want out of life. If an opportunity comes along but you feel unworthy of it, you won't pursue it. In fact, you may be blinded to scores of wonderful opportunities simply because of what you've heard from others about your worthiness to receive blessings.

Truth time: Do you honestly *believe* you're ready to move forward?

If not, identify the negative feelings and wrong beliefs you have and change them so they line up with the truth. (The truth is *never* that you're not good enough, by the way. You were made in the image of God. Who are you not to be *talented, creative, brilliant,* and *amazing?*)

For instance, you may need to know that you're not worthless. I can try to set you straight here, which would be lovely, but until you deal with this belief on a heart level, you can't really hear or embrace the truth and begin to live from that reality.

Negative, repetitive thought patterns can also impair your ability to move toward your best destiny. Have you ever heard a song that stayed stuck in your mind for the rest of the day? You don't need to be dancing to some tunes anymore. If your mind tracks are playing phrases or memories that disempower you,

you need to work on shutting them off. This is easier said than done, but some flower essence blends can help you with this.

Destiny Thieves

How many of the following potential-stealers are getting in *your* way? Each of these is followed by the flower essences that will help you overcome them.

- Guilt or shame from the past (Hyssop, Wormwood)
- Lack of confidence in your abilities (Buttercup, Lovage, Missouri Primrose)
- Unable to identify with success (Elecampane, Missouri Primrose)
- Pressed for time (Speedwell, Horseradish)
- Fear of risk (Borage, Black Currant, Lovage)
- Inability to handle stress (Lemon Balm, Pussy Willow)
- Lack of focus (Habanero, Comfrey)
- Fear of shame or humiliation (Hyssop, Borage)
- Fear of rejection (Oregon Grape, Black Currant, Malva)
- Procrastination (Blackberry, Tansy)
- Inability to connect with others (Joe Pye Weed, Elecampane)
- Low self-esteem or self-worth (Missouri Primrose, Buttercup, Sunflower)
- Disillusionment or discouragement (Borage, Horseradish)

Here's a little challenge. Make a list of a few bad decisions and destructive or dysfunctional behaviors. Now find some quiet time, sit down, shut your eyes, and revisit your earlier decision-making process for each one. I guarantee you a negative feeling is somewhere in that.

Look for a *common* theme in the above exercise. It isn't necessary to dig up all your dirt. Just direct your attention to one or two emotions that you recognize as negative influences. Make a note of the emotions for future reference. They're clues as to which flowers you need to combat them when they come calling again. Fear, anger, lack of confidence, shame, old woundings, etc. are all terrible decision-makers.

Here's another testimony.

> In working with Freedom Flowers for about six months, I reached a higher understanding of my self-worth, which led to a chain reaction of life-changing decisions. I walked away from a ten-year addiction to marijuana, cold turkey. I gradually stepped away from smoking cigarettes as well. I then walked away from an abusive relationship. I sank into depression for a bit but came out of it with ease and began to experience joy and hope again.
>
> The essences helped me clearly see my value and identity. They then helped with the tough transition and gave me clarity on which direction to go. The essences helped when I began to sink into

depression and eased the hopeless and out-of-control feelings.

Seneca, your wisdom and insight into what essences to use for each emotional struggle is one of the greatest gifts offered to this world. Lives are changed for the better because of what you have to offer. ~ Julie A.

FLOWER ESSENCES AND
PHYSICAL HEALING

MY AUNT AUDREY died at 104 ½. She didn't die of anything serious. She was having minor surgery and never came out of anesthesia. Centurions (people who live one hundred years) have interested me for a long time as I have tried to sort out the reason for their longevity. You always hear of a particular people, like the Japanese Okinawans, who supposedly live long lives because they eat lots of sea vegetables—or is it soy? The Hunzas eat millet. Some cultures eat bugs; others eat monkeys raw. Some eat sausage every day, and some smoke, but they manage to stay in decent health and continue to live independently.

From what I can discern, the only common denominator they have is an easy-going attitude and/or deep spiritual faith, a sense of humor, and they don't get too bent out of shape about anything. It seems to be obvious to me that what you are eating isn't nearly as important as what's eating you!

Frequently, when I'm explaining what I do and what flower essences are, I am interrupted with questions like, "What do you have for headaches? Got anything for energy?"

Flower essences don't work like that. Some essences correlate with physical symptoms, but mostly, it isn't as simple as herbs that do this or help with that.

If you want an herb or a drug, flower essences will disappoint. But if you're looking for a novel approach that addresses root causes, this is it. For the person on a quest for more energy, we need to look at what's draining them. Are they burned out from working too much at a job that bores them? Is a long-term illness contributing to the problem? Are they losing sleep from worry? Are they mad at someone?

Flower essences heal the mind. When that happens, the body follows. Any of us who have used essences for a while have usually had some kind of physical healing that happened unexpectedly while we were cleaning up our emotional health.

Let's again underscore the basic idea here: Flower essences are frequencies, and emotions are frequencies.

Each of your organs emits a specific frequency. The frequencies of some lower emotions are very similar to the frequencies of some organs. This means that the frequency of a negative emotion can have an affinity to a specific organ in your body and will try to settle there. As long as that frequency remains in the organ, it will be susceptible to infection, fatigue, dysfunction, etc. For example, anger can affect the liver, and fear can go to the kidneys or bladder.

By addressing an underlying emotional issue, you give the sympathetic organ the opportunity to recover. But if you refuse to address the emotional issue, true healing can't happen. A great example of this is people with cancer. The surgeons operate and say they got it all, but later the cancer comes back. This leads us to wonder: Did the surgeons not get it all, or did the person not address the root cause?

Facing death has a way of forcing us to re-prioritize and set matters right. But wouldn't it be nice if we elected to respond to our internal cries for healing *before* our bodies forced the issue?

A couple of colleagues and I created a chart that lists ailments and correlates them with possible emotional causes. It's not an absolute guide, but it may give you a hint or a starting place to work from. You can download it from http://bit.ly/rootschart. However, it's not necessary for you to know what emotions are contributing to which current physical condition. Go after the emotional issues you're aware of and then witness how much physical damage falls away.

It's also important to recognize the function of your body parts. For example, when I go to the place where I last saw my Dad, my vision blurs slightly. Apparently, I still have some trauma to deal with. This symptom is also an indicator of stress, by the way. I read the book *Relearning to See* by Thomas Quakenbush.[4] The basic premise is that the muscles around your eyes hold tension, thus distorting your lenses. If you can learn to relax and rework your muscle memory, your vision will normalize.

Another type of association is the powerfully debilitating sayings we have internalized. "The weight of the world is on your shoulders" translated to back and shoulder pain. My upper back/neck pain is almost always relationship-related. Because I recognize this, the symptom has become an effective barometer regarding the health of my relationships, so I know not to bother going to the chiropractor until I address the relationship issues.

Here are additional sayings that aren't helpful: We call people "stiff-necked" or stubborn and then call them "a pain in the neck." There's being "stabbed in the back," feeling that someone doesn't have your back, or wishing someone would just "get off your back."

For those who believe in the power of words as I do, it's best not to verbalize phrases like these. Why? Because words have frequencies, too! They have the power to affect you and others on every level but *only* to the degree of the emotion that fuels those words. The emotions you attach to them carry much stronger frequencies than words alone. I don't believe this should be a matter of just buttoning your lip; you also will have to deal with these issues at the heart level.

What if I could show you that the beliefs in your heart out-weigh and outperform your spoken words in the realm of frequencies? What if I could prove that people involved in the Word of Faith movements and those using positive affir-mations, confessions, or whatever you want to call them, are actually causing more problems than they're solving? I believe I can.

Sometimes I use kinesiology (muscle testing) to determine a correct essence for someone. I always start by having the person make one true statement and one bald-faced lie so I can gauge how much pressure I need to use when testing them. The untrue statement causes them to literally fold under pressure: They become momentarily, discernibly, and demonstrably weaker. I don't believe muscle testing connects us to absolute truth as this isn't a divination tool. It's limited to finding truth as it pertains to that individual's body, their subconscious mind, and their core beliefs—or to *relative truth* or what they personally believe to be true. Core beliefs and known facts are two different things. Head knowledge doesn't equal heart knowledge and vice versa. This understanding can work for us and against us.

The common way of teaching you to speak thoughts into manifestation is to find your positive declaration and repeat it. The assumption is that if you say it enough, it drops into your heart so that you believe, and then you receive. The problem is that if you repeatedly say something you don't truly believe in your heart, you're causing *additional harm.* People who proclaim, "I am healed of cancer" without truly believing it may essentially be killing themselves faster.

"Truly I tell you, if anyone says to this mountain, 'Go, throw yourself into the sea,' and does not doubt in their heart but believes that what they say will happen, it will be done for them" (Matthew 11:23).

It's better to work on what you truly believe before you attempt speaking things into manifestation. It's also effective to find a partner with rock solid beliefs and have them speak over you on your behalf. Connecting with a person who has triumphed in an area where you are struggling is priceless. Imagine having someone wholeheartedly on your side, speaking life, healing, and encouragement into you day after day. Flower essences can do this for you. They can also help you heal the emotional destruction that caused your core beliefs to misalign in the first place.

You have to get in touch with your feelings to receive true healing. When you acknowledge what set you off, triggering negative feelings, and work through the issues with flower essences, you'll find that many of your physical problems resolve themselves.

A Stanford University Medical School research quote released in 1998 by Bruce Lipton, a highly respected cell biologist, reported that emotional distress is the cause of *at least* 95 percent of illness and disease. He says the remaining 5 percent is genetic and caused by stress somewhere within the ancestry of individuals.[5] This means that 100 percent of the time, disease has an emotional root. But 5 percent of the time, you inherited that *personal emotional root* too!

The concept of cellular memory is somewhat controversial within the scientific community.[6] Cellular memory means the cells in our body record the dramatic things that happen to us. Psychological trauma, addiction, depression, and more can be tied to cellular memories. An astonishingly high number of rheumatoid arthritis sufferers have had a traumatic experience in childhood.[7] (Trauma is such a huge issue that it's getting its own chapter later on. So stay tuned.) Suppressing destructive memories takes enormous energy— energy that your body needs to repair itself, work, and function in healthy ways.

Your body has priorities that govern the use of its available energy. The first functions that usually go on the cutting-room floor when your available energy plummets are your healing and immune functions. Cellular memories affect you whether or not you are conscious of them.

Your subconscious mind works by association. Images and situations can trigger responses in you based on suppressed memories. These can cause anxiety, depression, and anger even when you don't know why. The connection becomes even harder to trace due to the fact that you *inherit memories at the cellular level.*

As I drove across the United States when I was twenty, I arrived at the Mississippi River, only to experience flashing images of long-gone riverboats and various people. I palpably experienced profound feelings of coming home. This did not relate to my past life. But my ancestors had lived along the Mississippi. My genetic roots are planted there.

This can also happen with organ transplants. A murder mystery was even solved because an organ donor began having dreams about the murder of the person whose heart she received. Her mother took her to a psychiatrist who concluded she was witnessing the actual event. The police were given enough detail to convict the donor's killer.[8]

What this means is that your unsubstantiated phobia may not even be yours. Deal with your personal issues, and you'll make one heck of an organ donor!

That said, you don't necessarily need to understand everything in your subconscious. But availing yourself of a round of flower essences that addresses stored traumas and then dealing with recovered memories (yours or an ancestor's) through prayer or your choice of healing modality is a beneficial plan for most people. Flower essences allow you to deal more gracefully with the emotional effects you're aware of. There are essences for every emotional state; knowing the root cause of your emotional condition isn't mandatory.

If you're still not convinced about the connection between the mind and the body, let's take inventory. What happens when you stress out? If you're like millions of other hard-pressed humans, you stop eating as healthfully as you otherwise would because you don't have time, your stomach is in knots, or because junk food seems to be just the solution to help you feel better.

On a physiological level, your immune system becomes suppressed, your adrenals go into overdrive, your digestive system is less efficient, your breathing becomes shallower, your sleep is disturbed, your muscles tense up, and your PH level becomes acidic. This may sound as if I'm defining extreme stress, but even minor stress is capable of producing these changes in your body. Even if just your digestive system is not functioning optimally, you'll absorb fewer nutrients, your colon may get clogged, and toxins will start accumulating. At some point, you'll experience adverse symptoms whether you're minimally stressed or an emotional mess. The bottom line is that if you want to be healthy, make yourself happy. The best thing you can do for your body is to live from a place of peace, love, and joy.

Two additional testimonies from flower essence users follow :

> Thank you, Freedom Flowers, for my Recovery drops. Since the accident in June of 2012, I have had very little energy and been somewhat depressed. The pain I was suffering in my broken and impacted left wrist was keeping me on edge most of the time. It was a constant ache

and reminder that it had little range of motion or strength left.

After you sent the Recovery remedy, I began to take them right away. I used three drops several times a day in a glass of water (and still do) and after a couple of weeks, I began to feel more positive. It was amazing, really! It was subtle, yet I knew something was different. I began to feel more positive about the physical therapy for my wrist and was happier doing it because I finally experienced hope for improvement.

Not only have my attitude and frame of mind changed, but I am seeing very positive results in physical therapy. I feel the wrist is responding more quickly. I know it sounds strange, but it feels as though the wrist is working with me now instead of resisting the therapy. I feel that I am moving toward greater and more extensive improvement. I am feeling a sense of well-being again. Thank you! ~ Melody Paasch

I met the wise and lovely Seneca at a workshop our Aglow Lighthouse hosted in Mount Shasta. What a humble, loving, quick-witted soul sister. She created a custom blend for me to alleviate raging menopausal symptoms, as all the oft-prescribed vitamins, herbs, and tinctures had previously failed to help. Some even worsened the nastiness. Miserable doesn't begin to define the day-to-day suffering, let alone the blanket-flinging, sleepless nights.

Within the first week, I noticed better rest and was able to fall asleep in between the hot flashes, which had also lessened. The breast tenderness and lumps were gone, and I experienced noticeable cognitive improvement, a stabilized mood, and an uplifted outlook. After a month, I felt more hormonally balanced than I had in ages. All from *flowers*, ***flowers***—those life-giving beauties we grow, snip, sniff, arrange, and paint. Flowers have unique vibrational signatures that facilitate healing. "All things bright and beautiful" indeed.

Additionally, I've also alternated between the "Good Grief" and "Crisis Care" blends to assist with a range of stressful, challenging life changes, including a pending empty-nest. So a big thank you to our awesome Creator, Jesus, and his pioneering, petal-pushing daughter. ~ Ruthmarie Runnels

TRAUMA

AS WE'VE ALREADY DISCUSSED, resolving trauma is necessary for total healing. Going forward, let's cover a few more points about the inner workings of your head and heart when you're dealing with your experiences.

Early Childhood

During the earliest years of life, our experiences are hard-wired without being subjected to the logical judgment that happens later in life. For instance, a crying child can aggravate his overworked, tired mother who might react with anger, yelling, or spanking rather than comforting him. The child, unable to understand his mother's weariness and exhaustion, only learns that when he expresses his needs, he will experience pain. If the pattern continues, what he internalizes about himself and his needs may cause him to believe that repressing feelings is the proper course of action and that he no longer deserves compassion. Thus, his course will be set for future frustrating relationships.

Children are egocentric. It takes them years to learn that the world doesn't revolve around them. This is because for the first part of their lives, the world certainly *did* revolve around them, from their perspective! Completely helpless at first, their every need was taken care of, 24/7/365.

One problem with this errant belief system is that they believe, in the core of their beings, that whatever happens is because of their presence, existence, and influence. This is why so many children believe it's their fault when parents divorce even though grownups know this makes no rational sense. I felt personally responsible for every single family issue that occurred through my teenage years. This is a common mindset among children and teenagers.

As discussed earlier, your subconscious mind works by association. So whenever you get into a situation that is in any way like an original trauma, the past becomes present. You relive the drama of the original event, even if the current situation is a scaled-down replica of the original. And the greater the trauma, the more likely your subconscious mind will trigger a similar, earlier situation.

Worst of all, you'll revert to that age you were when the original trauma occurred. You might be thirty now, but you know how quickly you can act like a five-year-old when trauma triggers show up. Bystanders and loved ones struggle to understand how a grown, rational person can melt down before them, but this is what's happening. Feelings don't have to make sense. The point is the feelings will prevail.

And that's good news. Feel the way you feel without judging yourself. Trying to explain bizarre emotional responses to others will just leave you feeling ashamed, repressing stuff, forming wrong beliefs about why you are the way you are, and prompting attempts to change it all—even if you don't have a clue about how or where to begin the process.

The bad news is that your traumatic memories are holding you hostage. Your memories remain intact, perhaps lying low in your subconscious where you don't have to be constantly in touch with the agony. But they remain because your subconscious has decided that holding onto the memory will protect you from future hurt.

My husband and I had friends over and lit a fire in our fire pit. At the end of the night, we let the fire die down and sprayed it with the hose before going to bed. The next day, I went to work. My husband hosed down the coals again and dumped them in a plastic garbage can and put it in our shop.

Hours later, the shop went up in flames. He ran in with the fire extinguisher, but the fire hit the gas cans, the motor oil, and the kerosene as he entered. In the chaos of the explosion, he couldn't find the door at first, but he eventually did. And he was fine . . . for a while.

After about a month, PTSD symptoms appeared. He experienced severe anxiety at the slightest scent of smoke, and he became paranoid about electrical appliances, even though they hadn't caused the fire. I couldn't use the slow cooker because it would have to be on all day, and I had to be extremely careful not to burn anything on the stove. The PTSD escalated to the point where he insisted we had to move. I didn't understand how that could possibly solve anything.

Many nights, we sat up to discuss this matter. He would shake and rock as I did my best to serve as the voice of reason, which I now know is a futile process. This became the catalyst for me to embrace flower essences on a more serious level.

In a crisis situation like the one my husband went through, when something bad happens, even if it's not life threatening, your subconscious makes sure you will *never ever* let it happen again. You won't put yourself in that position or in any position that's even close to similar. Instead, you enter fight-or-flight mode to make sure you come out in one piece.

Again, the greater the trauma, the broader the range of similar situations your subconscious will include. When this occurs, you re-experience the original emotions in their original intensity. When the triggers manifested, my husband's dire need was to escape, even though current situations were minuscule when compared to the initial trauma.

And trauma can come from small, seemingly benign events. For example, a four-year-old boy is told to be quiet because it is impolite to interrupt when grown-ups are talking. There's nothing wrong with that; it's one of the earliest lessons in manners that children learn. But the logic of this particular child internalizes this lesson as "What I have to say isn't important. Nobody wants to listen to me. My opinions don't count. People who get to talk measure up. They matter. I don't."

Later in life, as a grade-school boy and teenager, this young man will shrink from participating in group events and projects. He will withdraw and won't speak up about what concerns him and become reclusive, stripped of all self-worth. Well-mannered and well-liked, it will take one-on-one conversation to draw him out and get to know who he is. Despite his deep longing to be heard, understood, and valued, he'll pull into a shell.

It's even tougher to understand repressed memories because you have no idea where a bizarre reaction is coming from. Most people will develop some kind of explanation for their behavior, even if it requires blaming others. We feel a deep-seated need to produce a logical explanation, so that we don't feel crazy. So we rationalize why we do what we do. Other times, we chalk up our behavior to a phobia. I still have no idea why I used to be afraid of street sweepers.

With flower essences, you don't have to know the reasons for your trauma and reactions. You can take essences to deal with trauma and, if something comes to light, great, then process through it. If not, trust that healing is happening anyway. Pay attention to your dreams during the process. Healing comes through dreams, sometimes bringing a resolution, sometimes just purging via a subconscious release.

Dreams can also alert you to issues that you didn't realize were hurtful, usually childhood stuff that the older, rational you doesn't consider a big deal. These are your opportunities to move through the experience in a healthier way. Some great flowers for trauma are Star of Bethlehem, Arnica, Comfrey, Fireweed, and Echinacea.

If you have a history of trauma, some friends and I wrote a book called *Broken to Whole: Inner Healing for the Fragmented Soul* that goes into this subject in much greater detail.

Here is another testimony about flower essences.

> A horrible event happened to me a couple of years ago. It was so traumatizing that I didn't think I would ever heal from it. After using flower essences for a couple of weeks, I already notice a huge difference! Life seems "lighter," and I am actually starting to enjoy it on a regular basis. Seneca has been wonderful in helping me use these essences. She sends out periodic newsletters that really help with what you are taking and help you understand the process of healing you are going through. I highly recommend flower essences to anyone who needs emotional healing from going through horrible events in their lives.
> ~ Cheri Waller

HOW TO CHOOSE AND USE
YOUR ESSENCES

I F YOU'RE LIKE ME, you've already flipped to the back, read some flower descriptions and picked out a great many essences that look useful. The trouble is narrowing down your options.

Remember the analogy in the first chapter about the tuning forks and frequencies? Working with too many different essences at once can cause a lot of internal noise! Think of it like playing chords on a guitar or piano: There are lots of notes that work well together, but there's a limit to how many notes you can play at the same time before it sounds like a confused mess.

Many people prefer to use a single essence at a time for this reason. Doing so delivers a clean resonance. Single note users say they can progress through just as many essences, using them singly in succession, as those of us who use combinations over a longer period of time.

I personally prefer, though, to use combinations of flower essences. Either way, you will deal with a learning curve because if you only use one, you have to be sure you've chosen the right one at the right time. In combination, you can experiment some. If one doesn't do it, the others will.

On the other hand, knowing how to combine essences in a way that doesn't create a cacophony of noise is a bit of an art in itself. I tend to use a single essence when I'm in a lousy mood and need to move forward and when I know I won't need a month's supply of it. Sticking a few drops of Sweet Cherry in my drink is far more convenient than coming up with a combination bottle to manage a little flare up.

To create an effective combo, you need to focus on the primary (main) issue you want to attack. If you start to deal with issues with your father and then throw in something for fear of heights and your tendency not to be a good listener, you won't effectively address any of the areas you're attempting to deal with. So decide what's bothering you most right now and use essences that help resolve it.

In general, you shouldn't be taking more than seven essences at a time and take less than that if you're building your own combos and are new at it. I have solid feedback from someone who takes one combo during the day and a different one at night, but she reports that she feels the effects immediately. Most of us aren't that sensitive, but you can give it a try. Permission is granted to break all my rules and experiment.

Some essences are a little bit rough when taken alone because their healing actions require them to pull out repressed emotions. You will end up confronting issues that you previously had no interest in facing. You'll recognize these as you read the flower descriptions, with anything that is cathartic or deals with old memories, repression, or is a catalyst for change. There is the potential for emotions and situations to get worse before they get better. These essences need to be paired with something strengthening and soothing, something that gives courage and confidence and grounds you in love.

Some of these cathartic essences (Black-eyed Susan, for example) are best used in conjunction with another form of therapy. The user will need a stable support system as he or she faces dark issues: someone they can lean on and/or a robust spiritual connection. Many times, when I'm creating combinations for people, I will withhold essences like these until they can work through the basic stabilizing essences first.

You never want to take a person who's on the edge and push them over. The root of their problem needs to be dealt with for total healing, but you can choose the timing. Sometimes you have to chase symptoms with the first round of flower therapy. Sometimes you need to go straight to the roots.

As a rule of thumb, I add a soother/builder-upper essence in each combo. Some of my favorites are Lemon Balm, Self-Heal, Moonbeam Coreopsis, and Lettuce.

How Much? How Often? And for How Long?

The bottle says to take four drops four times a day. This is only a guideline, but there are no hard and fast rules here. You simply want to introduce the new frequency to your body's energetic field throughout the day.

Most of the time, we want essences to work fast, so it's better to take them more times a day, especially in the first few days. Sometimes, though, the realizations come too fast and are a bit tough to face. In these rare cases, cutting back can be helpful. Here are a few tips to help you use your essences frequently.

1. You don't *have* to add them to water. Water is key: The energetic vibes from the flower will transfer to all of the water you add it to. (Remember, your body is 70 percent water.) You have to have water to be a carrier. I do drink pure water, but water is also in tea, coffee, beer, etc. Put a few drops in whatever you drink.

Personally, I use essences by adding four drops to all my drinks. This may mean I have a sixty-four-ounce water jug with four drops of essences, or it may mean a little cup of tea with four drops in it. Every time I take a sip, that's one dose. If I make a pitcher of lemonade, I put drops in the whole container so I don't have to think about it later. If somebody else drinks it, that's fine. I end up with lots of pre-dosed drinks hanging around the house, which makes it a cinch to take.

2. Spike your drinks in advance. If you make a jug of sun tea, put your essences in when you make it so that you won't have to think about it later. It won't hurt anybody else if they have some unless they're on their own essence blend. Then they might have too many frequencies going on at once.

I have one of those big mugs sold at gas stations, the ones that are advertised as keeping your drink cold for six hours. They aren't lying. It really works. I fill that with ice water, add a few drops of flower essences, and hit the road. It lasts me all day. Every time I take a sip, I'm getting a dose. It's the perfect solution for me.

3. For those who would rather not ingest essences, no problem. Essences can be used externally too. They can be dabbed on pulse points, acupuncture sites, and/or places of tension or injury on the body. They can be added to bath water or shaken up in a shampoo or liquid soap bottle. Dandelion in particular makes a good bath additive. If you want to avoid the alcohol used as a preservative in essences, external use is a great option. You just have to remember to reapply frequently.

4. You can add essences to your humidifier tank but this option can affect everybody in the room, so choose carefully.

5. You can also use spray mists. I see these sold on other sites from time to time. I'm skeptical. I think the humidifier has

finer droplets that stay in the air. I like to use mist directly on my skin if I'm going to use this method. All the aromatherapy people can concoct wonderful mixes with this idea, I'm sure.

Some ideas would be to use lavender flower water and add four drops of "Peaceful Sleep" to a mister bottle. It would be great for your face after you wash, and it would help you wind down for the night.

Alternatively, you can add essential oils to water and add essences, but you have to shake really well when you do this because oil doesn't disperse in water, which is why I prefer the floral waters. They're enormously healing in their own way.

Again, frequency of use is key. You have to have a method that is easy and convenient or you won't take them often enough.

6. Don't forget to take them! You can even open your mouth and squirt a couple of drops "straight down the hatch." Lots of people do this. I prefer to dilute it because it charges every bit of the water in your glass, which helps extend the bottle. Another drawback is that you have to remember to take it several times a day. In addition, you might not like the taste. It's not bad, but your kids probably won't like it. My dog loves it, however, in water or straight in her mouth.

Just a reminder: flower essences take immediate effect, but you'll probably need to take them for three weeks to a month to see real change. And if you're working on deep childhood wounds, you may be on one or more essences for the long-term.

Sometimes, you'll need to keep cycling back around to the same essence or blend. Other times, you'll take some essences for a short time and feel so far past that issue that you can't imagine that you ever felt that way at all. Things that are not as deeply rooted take less time to adjust. Occasional funky moods can be changed in minutes, where severe childhood traumas will take time and may take several different combinations of essences. It's all very individual.

When It Doesn't Work

Flower essences are usually effective, but transformation doesn't always happen for a few reasons.

1. It's a frequency thing: The whole premise of flower healing is counteracting negative emotional vibrations with the exact flower frequency that's needed to bring the system into tune. If you're already vibrating that flower's particular frequency or a close enough frequency that you can't tell the difference, then you are using the wrong flower. But it's nice to know that if you choose wrong, the worst that can happen is nothing.

2. Improper or inconsistent use: If it's not working for you, examine your methods. Are you only using it once or twice a day? Are you forgetting to use it? Do you need a better system? Operator error is the most common reason essences fail.

3. You're on overload: Are you totally overhauling your life? Did you just go through New Year's resolutions, and you're fasting, organizing, essencing, and so on to a point where

your life is in so much turmoil that there's no normal to judge by? Are you using too many essences or trying to target too many different issues? Essences work very subtly. When you are dealing with a lot of change, their action can be hard to detect, or your system might go into overload and shut down.

4. Resistance: Flower essences won't take you down any road you're unwilling to travel. You always have a choice. You can choose to be happy, you can choose to let go of negative emotions, *but you don't have to.* The essences just make it easier to do so. Flower essences won't overrule your druthers. Your consent is vital for the healing process.

When It Works too Well

Healing crises are generally not well addressed in the flower essence world. Some books or sites will make enough mention of them to terrify people, so I thought I would share some of my experiences along with others that I've witnessed.

First, let's remember that in the natural health world, the "healing crisis" is always a good thing. It means the treatment is working, albeit a little too well. Also known as a "Herxheimer Reaction,"[9] this traditionally occurs when the body tries to eliminate toxins at a faster rate than they can be properly disposed of.

The more toxic one's bodily systems are, the more severe the detoxification or healing crisis. This means you'll have a temporary increase in symptoms during the cleansing or detox process, which may be mild or severe. You may feel worse and conclude that the treatment is not working. But these reactions are actually signs that the treatment is working and that your body is going through the process of cleaning itself of impurities, toxins, and imbalances.

In the same way, you can go through an emotional Herxheimer of sorts. Essences are exactly the same, except you're cleaning out old hurts and emotional issues you've been hanging onto that aren't serving you well.

It can be painful to see these issues come to the surface and have your false fronts stripped away. If it gets too intense, stop for a couple days, let matters settle, and try again with less frequent doses. The other option is to look at what you're taking and try a different approach with new essences. Then come back to the troubling ones later when you feel stronger.

You don't have to have a healing crisis for essences to do their job. I would say 95 percent of the time, people don't experience anything negative. It's not really an issue you need to watch for. You simply need to be aware of the possibility so you don't get blindsided.

People are most likely to go through a healing crisis if they have blocked issues or if they are using a substance or activity as a way of coping and avoidance. Flower essences tend to make us to face issues that we don't like in ourselves or something that needs our attention rather than letting us continue to suppress or ignore the roadblock. If this type of issue is standing in your way of healing, flower essences *will* have you face it down.

What does *that* feel like? I've documented moodiness, crying, disturbing dreams, social withdrawal, the surfacing of old memories, physical symptoms (especially in the stomach), and/or an inability to focus on day-to-day work because these issues are taking precedence and being worked through. Flower essences shine light on the truth— and sometimes the truth hurts.

A customer was on a blend for the long-term and needed a refill. She mentioned that she'd just found out she had a half-sister. I knew that she had a poor relationship with her dad, and considering this new bombshell, I decided to add in Sunflower. The next day, she told me, "I don't think this Sunflower is right. I'm just not happy at all."

Being happy all the time is unrealistic, even with flower essences. The goal is to react *appropriately* to whatever comes down the pike. Most of us handle issues backward and suppress the major issues and then overreact to the small ones.

We took the Sunflower out of the blend, and she has it separately to take as soon as she feels ready to confront the issue.

Certain essences are known to be potential crisis servers. One of these is Black-eyed Susan, which is a deeply cathartic essence with a long history of use in treating emotional amnesia or those issues you've blocked out.

Why should you put yourself through un-blocking? The events that are never processed can manifest in other ways, including physical problems and negative patterns in your life.

For example, lots of kids grow up in abusive homes. The healthiest survivors of these homes say, "I'm *never* going to hit my kids," and they turn out to be good parents in spite of what happened to them during their upbringings. Others grow up with unresolved hurt and repeat the pattern with their own children. They may even remember what it was like to grow up in an abusive home, but they've blocked out the feelings and the specific details of how bad the abuse truly was. The hurt never really went anywhere; they just learned how to stop *feeling*.

I'll throw the spotlight on myself again. One year, I had overwhelming fatigue and was constantly fighting off a cold, even though it was summer. I knew something was wrong physically. I'm a health-minded person, and I just don't struggle with these types of issues. I was making a great effort to feel better to no avail. *What in the heck is wrong with me?* I wondered.

Since everyone else on the planet thought I had "a little stress problem," I decided to take some Black-eyed Susan with the intent of gaining some understanding so I could move on to another flower essence. As I took it, I found that there were details surrounding the death of a family member that were still bothering me. I had attempted to use logic to squelch these emotions: "Dead is dead, doesn't matter how. Let it go already."

Would you say that to a friend? I wouldn't say it to my worst enemy— but I said it to myself! While taking Black-eyed Susan, I realized what I needed to do for my closure and gave myself permission to be upset and process my grief. It helped!

Meanwhile, my naturopath doctor told me that lungs process grief. That accounted for my fatigue and immunity problems.

I decided to keep taking Black-eyed Susan to see if anything else came up. I had a dream revealing some trauma from age five involving my dog. I came home from school one day, and Mom told me to climb some place high if I didn't want to be slobbered on because Moose was coming.

Moose was a humongous German Shepherd mix with a drool problem. His feet pounded the floor as he looked for me, so I panicked, jumped on Mom's and Dad's bed, and crawled in the middle so he couldn't reach me. Moose, of course, jumped on the bed to reach me, so I kicked him in the face. He went blind, freaked out, and ran into every wall, hitting his head repeatedly, and died.

I was horrified.

I don't remember talking to anybody about what happened or anyone trying to comfort me or realizing that I might have felt responsible. My family circled around Moose, trying to calm him down before he died while I watched from a distant willow tree. I think they thought I was fine because

I wasn't bawling my head off like most five-year-olds would after such an incident.

I don't remember crying at all past the initial screaming for Mom when he was hitting his head. It wasn't like I blocked these memories entirely, but with Black-eyed Susan, everything was fresh again, and I could cry and look at the situation from a more mature perspective.

From these two incidents that Black-eyed Susan brought up, you can see that I was at maximum capacity for unprocessed grief and that I needed to work through some essences to facilitate a healthy grieving process.

I moved on to Onion essence. Later I had a sweet, sweet healing dream about sitting on the floor with my dog with our heads snuggled into each other and my fingers in his fur. My dad (who usually represents Father God in my dreams) was standing over us, smiling.

Do you want to know what healed trauma feels like? It's remembering the event without the emotional intensity that was formerly attached to the situation. It's being able to talk openly about it with no shame or guilt or crying and being able to identify with others who are feeling the same kinds of things.

HELPING ANIMALS WITH
FLOWER ESSENCES

ONE OF THE MAIN REASONS I got into flower essences is that I absolutely love animals, and there are so few ways you can help them with traumatic emotional and behavioral issues. I have been around plenty of pets with past trauma, so I was really excited to see flower essences work. Animals respond quickly to them.

They don't have the hang-ups that we have (resistance to change or challenges to our understanding of how flower essences work). I'm pretty sure my dog understands them better than I do!

Zoe

Zoe is my border collie/hound mix. I met her because she was wolfing down whatever doggie delicacies she could glean from my compost pile. She had escaped her former digs with a tight choke chain cutting into her ribs that gave her big sores. You could see every rib and her entire backbone, and she was cowering in fear.

We obviously had to help her. I brought her into the house, and she ate spaghetti while my husband looked for bolt cutters to remove the choke chain. She has experienced nothing but trauma and drama from day one. Her tail had been severed, and she has been run over by a vehicle at least once and shot. Needless to say, she had issues.

Squeaky toys were seen as threats. She would hide if you rolled a ball toward her at any greater velocity than a snail's pace. It was heartbreaking to watch.

One day, when she was cowering and shaking from some perceived danger, I realized that she was not gaining ground emotionally, although she was bouncing back physically. So I gave her a basic emergency flower essence blend. Due to her dire situation, I didn't dilute it in water. I wanted an instant fix.

I had to I wrestle her down, pry her mouth open, and shoot the emergency blend in. It took a second, then her whole expression changed. She thought about it for a minute and then wanted to see the bottle. I offered it to her. She poked it around a little and gave it a slurp.

Since then, she has been an excellent essence taker. She will lick it off a spoon, or I can drop some in her bowl, announce what I'm doing, and she'll come running and guzzle water. She's so good.

Many times, there is an owner connection to whatever problem an animal expresses. They're perceptive and pick up the issues their owners are going through.

Mirroring an owner's mien is called "sympathetic resonance" by animal behaviorists. In other cases, you can unknowingly be doing something to aggravate your pet's problem. For example, Zoe doesn't like loud noises, thunder, and guns. If I'm on guard after watching the weather report to be sure she doesn't freak out when the first thunderclap hits, Zoe will pick up on my anxiety and become anxious too. Then when thunder does hit, her built-up anxiety (from our mutual concern) multiplies so that when I come to hug and coddle her, she thinks, "Gosh, it must be bad" and shakes even worse. But if I can remember to remain calm and act as if what's about to happen will be fine, she's much better.

Zoe's sensitivity keeps her on the same flower essence my husband is on, she picks up whatever is going on with him and makes it her problem too. Whenever she acts up, I joke to Mike, "She gets it from you, you know." Yesterday, I heard him tell her, "I'm okay, so you're okay too." Moral of the story is that if something is haywire with your pets, look into your own actions and circumstances. (You can always share the flower essences.)

How to Use Flower Essences

The dosage is four drops in the water bowl, making sure to use fresh water every day. It's fine if other animals drink it too. Alternatively, you can rub the drops into their gums or ears or anywhere you can get it to the skin. Adding drops to wet food is another option. Birds might like to be misted with an essence water in a spray bottle. Cats do not.

Here are some essences that lend themselves to common animal issues.

Apple: This is strength-boosting for animals that are sick or recovering from an illness. Flower essences don't directly treat the physical, but they do help give a consciousness of health. Apple reassures the animal—that may have picked up hypochondria from the owner—that it will be okay. Apple also helps create a sense of robustness for the runt of the litter.

Arnica: This is for shock or trauma and is especially great for animals that have been beaten.

Chamomile: This helps some cases of nuisance barking. It is especially good for emotional upsets accompanied by stomach upset, gas, or vomiting.

Chicory: This is for possessiveness, clinginess, and attention seekers. For animals that follow you everywhere and throw fits when you leave. Also helpful with animals that purposely get into trouble merely so you'll pay attention.

(Owner behavior indicated here. A codependent relationship might exist between the animal and owner if the owner displays codependent behavior and encourages it in his or her animal.) Helps with over-protectiveness or animal mothers who don't wean their babies.

Comfrey: This is good during training. It helps animals retain information.

Dill: This is good for sensory overload, feeling overwhelmed, or confusion for pets. Handy during travel or for animals that don't adapt well to schedule changes. Assists with sensitivity, loud noises, and new environments.

Echinacea: This is helpful for animals that have experienced severe, severe abuse, such as animals missing body parts, or any animal with extreme issues.

Evening Primrose: This assists animals that were rejected by their mothers or had some other bad association or traumatic experience with their mother or if their mother was in a traumatic situation during her pregnancy.

Fireweed: This facilitates new beginnings after devastation, such as animals that have been rescued from traumatic circumstances. You can also externally mist on burns, rashes, or "hot spots."

Lemon Balm: This soothes restlessness, insomnia, terrors, and anxieties.

Lettuce: This calms younger animals that are generally hyper: bounce around, no attention span, or go nuts. This is how they play, but they sometimes they just need to settle down and relax. More likely, you need them to settle down and relax.

Moonshine Yarrow: This helps protect animals from absorbing your bad moods. Sometimes the pet, dogs especially, pick up on discord within a house and negativity coming from the owners.

Oregon Grape: This helps them trust again. Animals who expect cruelty have a hard time trusting you to be nice, even though you've never given them a reason to anticipate abuse. For those who cower when you move your feet too close or raise your voice for any reason.

Pear: This reduces panic, chaos, and fear of going to the vet or anything that upsets them.

Pearly Everlasting: This helps with separation anxiety. For animals who have been previously abandoned.

Plantain: This soothes a temperamental, grumpy animal that doesn't like others; facilitates acceptance.

Red Clover: This reduces hysteria, especially indicated for cats. Use it when taking an animal to the vet. If you have one fearful animal that riles up the others, they all need Red Clover. You can also use it as a preventative for triggering situations, e.g., when thunderstorms are forecast.

Self-Heal: This helps stimulate the animal's innate healing process and will to live.

Sow Thistle: This reduces bullying behavior either for the bully or the animal being bullied. Great for multi-pet houses.

Star of Bethlehem: This helps to resolve all kinds of trauma whether old or still fresh, physical, mental, or emotional. This is a great essence to start with when you rescue an animal and don't know its history.

Sweet Chestnut: This comforts animals that have given up the will to live. For those who deal with self-mutilation or starvation. For wild animals now in captivity or animals rescued from a factory farm.

Sweet Pea: This instills a sense of home and family. When you bring an animal home or move to a new place, Sweet Pea helps pets transition. Also great for dogs who don't stay home.

Teasel: This comforts pets who have become depressed after witnessing fighting and arguing between family members.

Tiger Lily: This calms hostile or aggressive animals.

White Chestnut: This reduces obsessive behavior, restlessness, and helps animals that seem preoccupied.

Wild Rose: This decreases resignation and apathy, restores the will to live, and is good to use with a long-term illness or with animals that don't seem interested in life.

Violet: This minimizes shyness when a pet would like to be sociable and longs to be friends but can't.

Yarrow: This reduces environmental sensitivity and helps an animal to be less affected by the moods of others, including their owners.

Freedom Flowers Pet Blends

These are convenient pre-mixed essences to deal with specific issues available at http://bit.ly/petblends.

Anti-Aggression flower essence addresses fear-based aggression, bullying behavior, hostility, underlying trauma, snapping, chewing, biting, and resource guarding.

Anti-Separation Anxiety promotes a feeling of calmness and security while you're gone.

Crisis Care is helpful in emergencies, accidents, vet visits, or any circumstance that provokes a meltdown.

Focus is very helpful during the training stages. Helps them with memory and staying on task.

Harmony brings cooperation to multi-pet households, especially involving different species. Helps everyone stay calm and get along. Especially indicated when a new pet is joining the clan.

Indoor Pet helps those who don't get enough outside time to stay healthy and grounded. Not a substitute for outside time but will help.

New Home helps your pet adapt to new family, home, or other changes.

Peace for Pets helps animals that have anxiety or phobias. Especially intended for fireworks and thunderstorm season.

Recovery for Pets is supportive and strengthening during illness or post-surgery. It gives them hope and reassurance that they are on the mend and gives them an overcomer mentality.

Trauma-Free is ideal for rescue animals, pet shop purchases, or any pet when you're not sure of their history. It helps them get over their past and learn to trust and feel secure.

The following testimony shares how flower essences helped a dog.

> My friend's dog just had puppies about six weeks ago. She developed a bad skin infection on top

of nursing puppies. The vet gave her antibiotics last week, but the dog kept getting worse. As of yesterday, she had lost all the hair on her back end. My friend said her skin was so red that it looked as if someone had taken a blowtorch to her. I gave her some of my "Crisis Care" to try first. I thought maybe it would jump start her healing. She just came in and asked what I had done to her dog. She said her dog dove into her water bowl and downed the whole thing. This morning she said almost all of the red was gone except for one small pink spot! ~ Michelle Hill

Q & A

How will I know it's working? What changes should I expect?

You can expect the following:
- new realizations
- pertinent dreams
- changes in the way you look at situations
- changes in the way you see yourself
- peacefulness
- a positive outlook
- a release of accumulated tension
- the ability to remember a formerly painful event with a sense of peace and closure
- Flower essences don't affect you the way conventional medicine does. Expect subtle changes. They don't overhaul your personality. They don't change you into anything but your most positive self.

What happens if I use the wrong essence?

Nothing. Unlike homeopathic medicines, there are no potential bad reactions. The essence simply won't work. If you're having trouble, we have a customized combo we can give you, which includes a brief consultation. We'll help you find what you need.

Isn't it just a placebo-effect working?

I suppose that could be part of it, but the placebo effect doesn't explain why my dog and so many other animals I work with have had such positive responses. In addition, children and others who don't understand what's being given to them often have the most dramatic results.

Are they safe?

Yes! Babies, pets, elderly people on all kinds of medications—anybody can take these. Energy medicine is the only area of health care where there has never been a documented case of harm.

The only issue for some might be the little bit of alcohol used as a preservative, but it's minuscule. You could add the essence to hot tea and let the alcohol evaporate, or dot it on your pulse points or areas of tension. There is also no possibility of overdose.

Q & A

I don't know where to start.

Start with what is bothering you most. Get a handle on daily life and then go deeper. Most problems in life are connected. Essences are multi-functional, so you'll probably have more healing than you anticipate, even if it's not something you notice right away.

I believe everyone should do a round of trauma-releasing essences at some point. A good time to do this is when you don't have a lot of other turmoil happening in life and you have a good support system of family and friends in places. If you're not there yet, use essences to address your daily stressors.

It's easiest and most cost-effective to start with a pre-mixed blend. If none are the right fit, you can get a customized blend from a flower-essence practitioner. You can also buy individual flower essences that are right for you and use up to seven of them together at a time.

Should I quit taking medicine? Will it interfere with prescriptions or over-the-counter drugs?

No. Flower essences are the perfect adjunct to whatever it is you are doing. There is zero possibility of a drug interaction. As you begin to feel better, you can work with your doctor for adjustments to your medication.

My friend/spouse/coworker would benefit from essences but doesn't want to hear about it. Should I just spike his or her drink?

No. Don't do it. Respect the person's choice. It can be tempting, and your heart may be in the right place, but it's still wrong. A secondary piece of advice is that you can take essences to deal more effectively with a person who is being difficult if that is an issue. Sometimes, just becoming your best self rubs off on those around you, and they decide to go ahead and try flower essences because of the noticeable effect they've had on you.

How do we know what all the flowers do?

A starting point for this information is by an ancient method now known as the Doctrine of Signatures. It is unclear when this originated, but we have writings that hint at 131–200 AD. But Jacob Boehme finally outlined a clearer system, usable by plant people centuries later, in his book, *De Signatura Rerum (The Signature of All Things.)*[10]

Jacob had a spiritual experience, revealing the simple concept that God marked everything He created with a sign. This sign points us to how we can use it for the purpose it was intended. He was promptly kicked out of town based on the advice of the pastor there (the mark of any juicy revelation) but later allowed to move back home provided he did not write any more books. (He failed to comply, but I digress.)

In order to understand a flower's actions, we can observe the following: overall appearance, habitat, color, flower shape, growth habit, unusual characteristics, and names. *Doctrine of Signatures* rarely gives us the whole story. Rigorous testing is still needed to confirm the action and to develop a greater, more specific understanding.

As you're discovering here, essences have made a huge difference in my own and in my clients' lives. It's amazing how much freedom can come in little blue bottles. It's amazing how something so simple can cause so much change.

I invite you to explore essences for yourself and push the limits on what you think you can heal from, move toward, and leave behind.

FREEDOM FLOWERS A–Z

All of these are available as individual essences or in combinations if marked as such at www.freedom-flowers.com.

Angelica flower essence helps us to remove any notions or hang-ups we might have that tell us we need an intermediary between us and God. If we have set a person or a religious system as a substitution for a direct line of communication to God, Angelica shows us how we've done so and that this is not necessary. Find it in our "Open Ears" blend.

Apple is an encourager that helps you make healthy choices. Apple counteracts health-related fears, such as the fear of cancer returning or hypochondria (however mild it may be) but does so in an empowering way rather than by denying prudent actions you need to take to ensure health. Apple inspires a positive outlook throughout the recovery process, which is healing in and of itself. Apple is helpful any time you need to regain the balance between body, mind, and spirit. Find Apple in our "Recovery" blend.

Apricot helps us step into new seasons in our lives as if we were born ready. It can also help you to be sensitive to the subtle clues that everything is about to change and how to best position yourself to be the first to reap the rewards. Use Apricot anytime you sense being in transition, especially if you're feeling apprehensive.

Arnica helps deal with emotions that are locked in the body after accidents or violent experiences. Arnica is the remedy of choice for dissociative disorders, puzzling illnesses, or autoimmune diseases that don't respond to other methods of treating the physical symptoms. Arnica is also helpful for use immediately after accidents to release the shock held in the body's musculature. Alternatively, it can be used as a release of old, locked-in emotional or physical trauma. Find it in our "Align," "Fragment Finder," "Crisis Care," and "Aftershock" blends.

Aurinia instills a deep security and trust that you are taken care of and that you have already been given everything necessary to succeed in the place you're called. Dreams, visions, and other avenues of spiritual awareness help to build a resolve of boldness and fearlessness. It helps us feel not just more equipped but also eager to tackle tasks put off for fear of different reasons/lies. Over-responsibility based on insecurities level out to a confident, balanced way of working. Find it in our "Prosper" blend.

Basil helps to restore the sacred aspect of sexuality. It can be used wherever there has been objectification, degradation, or abuse, whichever side of it you were on. Basil helps to shift the perspective from a purely physical act to one of the deepest expression of intimacy. Use Basil if there are any shame or negative feelings toward sex. Find it in our "Healthy Intimacy" blend.

Bear Grass clears energetic blockages in the spine. Beneficial for nerve-related spinal injuries, back problems in general, and headaches. Bear Grass can also be a bit of an awakener, bringing creative ideas and dormant talents to the forefront, as well as dealing with some of the attitudes that are not serving us well. This is not always a comfortable situation for the short term, but the long-term effects of changing your thinking and your way of operating that align with your particular gifts are so worth it! Find it in our "Align" blend.

Bee Balm is an explosive little energy generator. It ignites passion that we need to carry on with projects or goals and helps us find joy and inspiration in the day to day. Bee Balm gives you something to look forward to while helping you enjoy the moment you're in. Find it in our "Ignite" and "Joy" blends.

Bird's Foot Trefoil helps with emotional eating, binging, bulimia, and anorexia. It helps us understand the pain in the lives of those who put us down. Find it in our "Craving Control" blend.

Bittersweet's tendrils reach out in the spirit to pull in and grab hold of parts of us that have been lost or hiding in the shadows. It imparts a courageousness to go deep into the dark places, facing our fears and nightmares to do a spiritual "jail break." If you do any kind of journey work or spirit travel, Bittersweet is an ally in seeing in the dark, and will also help you "allow" these kinds of experiences to happen. Buy it individually or in our "Fragment Finder" blend.

Blackberry releases breakthrough. Blackberry is great for the person with lots of ideas and little ability to carry them out. It helps translate grand schemes into specific plans of action. Blackberry vines push up through rocks and hard earth; they are all about the breakthrough! Blackberry will also have you speaking up for what you want and what you feel is right. Blackberry enables a beautiful balance between too timid and too forceful in speaking your truth. Find it in our "M&M" and "Vision Quest" blends.

Black Currant deals with a plethora of fear-based issues: fear of risk, fear of change, fears of abandonment and death, or just unexplained general fears and anxiety. Those who have trouble moving forward in life or who can't let go of the familiar to take hold of something new can benefit from Black Currant. In particular, it seems to address the fear of non-existence, which can be helpful with parts work. Find it in our "Stay Calm" blend.

Black-eyed Susan is the classic anti-repressor. It is a powerful essence for unlocking areas of old trauma or painful areas that we've walled off ourselves. Black-eyed Susan lends us the courage to go deep within and release what has been trapped in our subconscious. This essence will bring light into the darkest areas, helping you to identify and shed hurts and burdens. Find it in our "Fragment Finder" blend.

Black Locust is protective against energy that is projected deliberately. When we are vulnerable to attacks from others and can feel their anger and negativity intentionally directed at us, Black Locust is strengthening. Find it in our "Yarrow Shield" blend.

Bleeding Heart is for heartbreak and codependency. It helps release painful emotional attachments and restores balance, helping you live and love with your whole heart, not from brokenness and neediness. A great essence to take when a relationship ends, whether it is from a breakup, death, move, or desire to break a cycle of codependency. Find it in our "Good Grief" and "Heart Healer" blends.

Blue Vervain is a must for those who deal with tension in the neck, shoulders and upper back and mitigates the effects of stress coming from mental exertion and focus. Emergencies, deadlines, and intense focus on the task at hand for too long of a period can set you up physically for a stress response. Blue Vervain, in time, will help you develop a more balanced way to be successful. It is essential for the workaholic. Find it in the "Align" blend.

Borage is excellent to lift heavy hearts and encourage the user. Its action is strengthening and supportive of change, allowing one to trust in higher guidance. It imbues optimism, gladness, courage, and enthusiasm. Borage should be used for any situation that is difficult to face or when you're feeling disheartened or discouraged. Borage is a great heart remedy, opening you to feel greater levels of love and compassion. Find it in our "Joy," "Good Grief," "Tomorrow," and "Menoblend."

Boxwood helps you break free of the expectations of others. This essence can help those who feel they have had certain behaviors trained into them, especially if they have been overly compliant to fit into the "box." If you had a strict upbringing with a very strong sense of what kind of behaviors, thoughts, and opinions are acceptable, Boxwood can shift you into less shameful states of consciousness. You can still mind your p's and q's, fitting into situations and different company with Boxwood while standing your ground where your individuality matters. Find it in our "Bravely You" and "Peak Performance" blends.

Bull Thistle helps release negative past experiences with structure or authority, allowing you to see situations more clearly and trust healthy structure and leaders. This essence also helps ease fears of being controlled or confined. It is a solid essence to address claustrophobia and for those who use their authority too strongly for fear of losing control.

Buttercup helps those who are frequently overlooked to shine forth with full consciousness of their unique gifts and abilities. Buttercup inspires you not to judge yourself based on conventional ideas of achievement or by comparing yourself to others but to realize your worth based on who you are not on recognition from others. This is also a helpful essence for those who have to step into a phase that, by some standards, would be considered a less important path. Buttercup shows you how you are successful at whatever stage you're in. Find it in our "Confidence," "M&M," "Vision Quest," and "Peak Performance" blends.

Butterfly Weed helps with fear of commitment, frigidity, impotence, or sexual obsessions. It aids a multitude of relational issues that boil down to control, boundary issues, and losing interest when situations become difficult, mundane, or too emotionally intimate. Butterfly weed helps us to reach a deeper level of relationship. Find it in our "Healthy Intimacy" blend.

Calendula fosters warm, sensitive communication in those who tend to speak harshly. Those who are too blunt can find better ways of communicating what needs to be said without shredding the other person. It also helps us to recognize the creative nature of our words and therefore is an aid to writers, speakers, teachers, and prayer warriors. Calendula is especially indicated during relationship work and for anyone whose livelihood depends upon their ability to communicate with warmth and compassion.

California Poppy helps those looking for their true spiritual path. It helps navigate between false spiritual experiences and man-made religious systems to find a real connection from within your own heart. It also helps with the compulsion to buy new things, gamble, feed addictions, or other attempts to fill a hole in one's heart. California Poppy helps inner development so you can move into advanced states of spiritual experience without being pulled in a direction that serves somebody else's purpose. Find it in our "Open Ears" blend.

Camas helps right and left brain hemispheric balance . It reconnects neural pathways, clears obstacles and negativity, and is especially indicated for autism, stroke recovery, communication issues, focus, grounding, and sound healing. Find it in our "Focus" blend.

Catalpa is a deep heart healer that can be effective either for present wounding or old childhood pain that persists. This one is especially indicated for any type of abandonment, betrayal, or feelings of being unloved. For children and adults who are going through divorce or separation or dealing with a death, Catalpa is a comforter and a reassurance that they are worthy of love and that love is a force they can never truly be separated from. Find it in our "Heart Healer" and "Good Grief" blends.

Chamomile helps with stress that manifests physically in the stomach. A great essence for stress-related digestive disorders, chamomile is helpful with a variety of childhood dramas, from mysterious upset tummies, colic, fussiness, and crying. Chamomile is a super soother. For children who insist on being held, throw tantrums, and want everything and nothing, chamomile is the remedy. It encourages a brighter, sunnier disposition. It also helps with emotional tension related to PMS and menstrual stress. Find it in our "Good Grief" and "Aunt Flo's Secret Weapon" blends.

Cherry Plum guards against breakdown, out-of-control episodes, and bad decisions made in desperation. It helps users to express emotions they fear in healthy, non-destructive ways and remain calm and rational in difficult situations where they would otherwise explode or come apart. Cherry Plum makes it easier to access spiritual insight that you will use to overcome emotional situations. It also helps you trust that you have divine guidance. Find it in our "Crisis Care" and "Craving Control" blends.

Chicory flower essence is for those who feel deprived of love, those who want to be surrounded by those they care for and may tend to fuss over them. Chicory helps with abandonment issues and wounds from rejection that result in holding people so tightly that they pull away, creating a vicious cycle. Chicory helps you love deeply and completely without any strings attached. You're able to give generously to others while genuinely expecting nothing back. You keep healthy boundaries with others, allowing them to walk their own path. You fulfill your own needs and give from a sense of abundance. It brings a sense of security in all close relationships, and once those close to you feel the release, they, too, are free to love with no reservations. Chicory flower essence is indicated for children who demand attention or who are crying, clingy, or throwing tantrums. Chicory teaches about love; it calms neediness by revealing the source of unconditional love—and with that comes new-found security. Find it in our "Heart Healer" blend.

Chrysanthemum fosters a sense of positive, enduring energy throughout the day and helps bring a better alignment of the spirit in relationship to the body and soul. Typically, the spirit is suppressed, and since it has a direct line to God and wisdom for life and healing, it's to our body's and soul's advantage when it has a more prominent place in our lives. Chrysanthemum seems to mitigate the soul's concerns about letting a radical spirit have its place and a more harmonious tri-unity can emerge. Find it in our "Recovery" blend or as part of the Body Coaching program.

Coleus helps increase dream recall. Just as the coleus doesn't need sunlight to be vivid, you don't need the daylight to see clearly about any of the following: your destiny, your hang-up, your potential for averting disasters, or seizing new opportunities. Coleus increases the vivid pictures waiting in the shadows. Find it in our "Dream Drops" blend.

Comfrey reverses the effects of old traumas that have caused you to shut down in an attempt to protect the conscious mind. Its repair of the nervous system can bring about beneficial effects on memory and the ability to receive information through dreams and other avenues of spiritual awakening. It may stimulate dormant or atrophied areas of the brain to become more active. Since the nervous system is the bridge between mind and body, you may also experience better coordination, better blood pressure, improved digestion, and accelerated healing from broken bones or surgery while taking comfrey. Find it in our "Dream Drops," "Focus," "Fragment Finder," and "Aftershock" blends.

Coreopsis reduces cravings and combats addiction and depression. It also ups your sense of confidence, strengthens you, and helps you deal with stress. Coreopsis is in our "Smoke-Free" blend but lends itself well to food issues and is in our "Craving Control" blend as well.

Cosmos helps us to translate abstract or emotional concepts into clear speech. It's helpful for those who try to communicate matters of a spiritual nature that are not always easily translatable into practical language for the average listener. It's also helpful for those who become overexcited and the words come out in a jumble or for those who recognize the difficulty and resort to an overly simplified statement that lacks the depth and intricacy needed to properly communicate the issue. For those who lack focus or are overwhelmed when trying to communicate, Cosmos helps bring the subject down to a level where it can be articulated. By extension, as the individual grows more confident in their self-expression, more of the personality can connect with the higher mental function and be expressed more fully.

Daffodil increases sensitivity and connection to the voice of Creator. Daffodil facilitates illumination and clarity when facing complicated decisions and identity crises and is the perfect adjunct to spiritual pursuits. It relieves feelings of shyness for those who can't find their voice or who are afraid to use it. Daffodil helps you see the big picture and realize where you fit into it. The big-picture view becomes necessary when we become fixated on an object of desire or, conversely, something we dislike. Both extremes become a stumbling block to receiving undistorted and unbiased communication from a higher source. Daffodil also helps cut through negative communications in earthly relationships. Its clarifying action helps you to truly hear what's being said or not said, allowing you to deal with the real issue. Find it in our "Open Ears" blend.

Dandelion works out the knots and stress in muscles. For the hard-driving enthusiastic personality that pushes beyond their physical capacity to carry out intense activity, dandelion will tune you in to what your body needs and help you process much-needed inner quiet time. If you tend to throw yourself full on into too many activities, over-plan, or over-schedule, Dandelion is a great balancer for a more sustainable lifestyle. Find it in our "Stress Less" and "Align" blends.

Datura also aids with spiritual vision and cuts through illusion and works through dreams as well. It makes it easier for you to let go of old ways and increases your faith to step into the new and unknown. Find it in our "Dream Drops" and "Vision Quest" blends.

Dill deals with sensory overload. Our present culture tends to distract and over stimulate to the point where we have a type of spiritual ADD. There are retreats for this sort of thing, but the trick is to remain functional in a modern world where sights, sounds, and smells from every direction constantly bombard us. The usual means of coping is to become hardened so we don't become overwhelmed. But what's needed is to refine and clarify what we are sensing so our senses become a vehicle for revelation. Dill helps put it all together to discern the whole picture rather than a bunch of sensory impressions. Sometimes, when your dream life is too fragmented to form a coherent thought, sensory overload is indicated. Dill flower essence can free up your dreams from overload so they can be better used as means of revelation. Find it in our "Dream Drops" and "Yarrow Shield" blends.

Double Delight Rose helps us let go of the struggle of our logical mind being able to accept a paradox and grab onto a counter-intuitive path or way of being. The process of getting out of your own way isn't as simple as these statements, however. If you have been in a long-term struggle to apprehend and work out a paradox in your life, Double Delight can help. With Double Delight, you may find yourself transitioning to a place of happiness that you've thus far been unable to accept. Double Delight can also resolve generational trauma, trauma that you feel but that never happened to you. When you resolve an issue in the place of your ancestor, you free yourself and also your descendants from wounds and hardships that never should have been theirs to deal with. Use Double Delight for closure and the release of family, racial, or cultural trauma.

Easter Lily addresses the spiritual and physical aspects of the reproductive organs, especially in women. It helps when there has been abuse or misuse of sexuality, even on a generational level. This trauma can linger in the reproductive system, causing more issues than should be normal. For this reason, Easter Lily is helpful for women whose experience of menopause is difficult. This is also a very helpful essence for any woman who needs or has undergone a hysterectomy. Find it in our "Menoblend, " "Healthy Intimacy," and "Aunt Flo's Secret Weapon" blends.

Echinacea helps transition from an old traumatized self-image to the new fully-integrated person. It maintains a protection around you while you are in a vulnerable weakened state, but doesn't leave you there. Childhood traumas can shatter a person's core identity, causing you to dissociate or adopt a different persona for survival. Echinacea helps restore true identity and wholeness by releasing the old, especially for those who do not feel fully present. Find it in our "Menoblend," "Fragment Finder," "Floral Defense," and "Aftershock" blends.

Elder stimulates the recovery process by building joy, energy, and resilience and is an emotional decongestant. It relieves stagnant, heavy emotional states and replaces them with peace and a strong sense of optimism. Elder also instills a sense of beauty and youthfulness. It's a rejuvenator and strengthener for those who are "feeling their age." It also calms fears and helps you realize your inner strength. Find it in our "Recovery" blend.

Elecampane helps those who feel out of touch with the general population. It helps you be comfortable being yourself in social situations and also enhances self-worth. It brings a stronger sense of individual identity and helps you integrate new information and experiences. Find it in our "Confidence" or "Bravely You" blends.

Evening Primrose helps heal emotional pain absorbed from the mother in early childhood. It is especially recommended for those who were adopted or unplanned, causing stress in utero. It's also indicated for mother issues, such as being over-controlled or used to boost her self-esteem or to fulfill her ambitions. You had to be a model student or excel in music, dance, sports, or another area. It opens the ability to form deep, lasting relationships by dealing with issues of rejection; fear of commitment and parenthood; and difficulties dealing with sexual and emotional feelings. It promotes healing of early childhood trauma and helps users develop greater emotional intimacy with others. Find it in our "Peak Performance" and "Healthy Intimacy" blends.

Feverfew supports change and helps regulate hormonal disturbances. It brings out strength and tenacity and instills calmness, softness, and serenity. Find it in our "Menoblend" and "Aunt Flo's Secret Weapon" blends.

Fireweed is about springing up from the ashes with new passion and purpose after devastation. It is the first plant to grow after forest fires and other severe disturbances and is a great remedy for burn out. Its action helps you recover your true purpose in life and can help you clear out old habits, behaviors, and armor that aren't serving you. Fireweed is about restoration on the deepest level, supporting an immediate rekindling of vitality. Find it in our "Crisis Care" and "Aftershock" blends.

Fleabane is for those who suffer from depression and negative thought patterns. It uplifts and brings clarity, lightness, openness, cheerfulness, and a positive desire for change. It is a bit similar to Yarrow in that it helps seal us up where we've been too porous and vulnerable, but its action focuses more on protection against the undertow of sadness, pessimism, and hopelessness. Find it in our "Joy" blend.

Gaillardia's essence is that of a survivor. Part firewheel plant, part security blanket, Gaillardia helps us shift from a recent blow or trauma to peace, comfort, and focus via a quick regrouping to a new path. Unlike some essences that almost have an "erasing" quality, Gaillardia doesn't make light of what you've been through. Instead, Gaillardia seems to empower you to stand unwavering in the face of opposition or trials with strength.

Goldenrod instills self-trust and confidence, especially in those who don't have a strong sense of their individual identity. A key to identifying this type of personality is when the individual modifies their behavior to fit their present company. We cannot help but derive our identity, value, and meaning from external sources; however, Goldenrod will help increase personal affirmation and attention. It helps one to stop seeking peer approval and gain inner strength and conviction about who they truly are. This is a great essence for the teen years when identity is shaky and peer pressure is strong. Find it in our "Confidence," "Peak Performance," and "Bravely You" blends.

Golden Yarrow is for the social and mental aspects of relating to others without feeling vulnerable. It helps you to interact with others from a place of strength combined with sensitivity. It's especially good if you are putting up walls in relationships with other people. Find it in our "Yarrow Shield" blend.

Habanero brings clarity when there is mental fogginess, absentmindedness, forgetfulness, or an inability to focus. It does this by clearing out repressed trauma, which results in a greater flow of energy throughout the body and a mental awakening. This essence may require you to process some issues that you have suppressed in the past. Find it in our "Focus" and "Ignite" blends.

Harebell's lesson is that you are good enough just as you are, worthy of your Creator's unconditional love, and to stop seeking love in the wrong places and compromising who you really are in order to get love. It helps you allow things to fall into place by resting in faith rather than trying to force things to happen. Harebell also helps those who have a hard time opening their heart to others. By receiving true and pure love from the Source, you can let it flow freely to others. Find it in our "Confidence," "Bravely You," "Heart Healer," "Powerhouse," and "Peak Performance" blends.

Horseradish puts you back in the driver's seat. You *can* move forward and change direction. Feeling stuck? Feeling like a victim of circumstances? Feeling frustrated or fearful? Horseradish powers through all that. You'll have to take responsibility for your situation, but Horseradish will build you up, fire you up, and move you out of your current rut by dislodging fear, low self-esteem, and blame-shifting. Find it in our "M&M," "Powerhouse," and "Ignite" blends.

Hyssop addresses guilt and shame-based issues and all their cousins: self-sabotage, self-blame, fear of being judged, perfectionism, and unworthiness. Hyssop works within the structures of thinking we've built and reverses the internal judgment and self-condemnation we fall into. Some degree of judgment is necessary but not as a constant state where you dwell. This kind of self-punishment creates a barrier toward receiving the blessings in life. Hyssop is especially wonderful for those who grew up in a guilt-based religious system that has become a stumbling block to a true relationship with Creator. Find it in our "Healthy Intimacy" and "Prosper" blends.

Iceberg Rose helps to heal the effects of sexual abuse or harassment and restore a sense of purity and innocence. This essence encompasses all ages and genders but seems especially useful for children, who can be sensitive even to an illicit intention. Adults who experience frigidity or lack of emotional involvement connected to sex can benefit from Iceberg Rose, whether they recall an abusive situation in the past or not. Find it in our "Healthy Intimacy" blend.

Indian Paintbrush is a stimulator of creativity, passion, vision, and self-expression. It's useful to jump-start the creative process but also to see it through. It helps us to meet our own needs during intense times when we tend to overlook basic self-care, such as eating and rest because we are busy doing our thing. We are all creative beings whether we consider ourselves artists or not. Indian Paintbrush will sustain you in your creative journey. Find it in our "Ignite" blend.

Joe Pye Weed resolves issues connected to resistance to solitude, for it is when you are alone that you meet God. If you're the type of person who needs to have the TV, phone, or other electronic device on all the time, Joe Pye can help you be more comfortable and receptive during the quiet times. Many spiritual experiences exceed the comprehension of the deductive mind. This can cause fears, blocks, and avoidance to spiritual practices on conscious and unconscious levels. Joe Pye eases the resistance to moving toward the unknown and allows an assurance of safety to surface. The types of fears that Joe Pye confronts are fears associated with kidney and bladder problems, so it has a cleansing and stimulating effect on these organs. Other benefits to taking Joe Pye Weed are healthier friendships with others. Find it in our "Dream Drops" and "Open Ears" blends.

Kerria helps balance and stabilize emotions, especially in cases of excessive mood swings and rage. It helps to counter polarized moods, bringing a healthier sense of self and personal power. Find it in our "Anger Management" blend.

Klip Dagga is calming, strengthening, and adds will power to the person struggling with addiction. Its Latin name *Leonotis* is after a lion, and a lion is the essence disposition. It helps you face problems head on with the heart of a lion.

Larkspur flower essence is great for leaders. It helps with the dualistic yet often unbalanced or opposing roles of the magnanimous charismatic side and the humble, inspiring servant-leader. Larkspur helps you orient and ground your values into the way that you lead and express your mission to encourage and inspire others.

Lavender flower essence helps quiet the mind. It helps you learn to balance your mental, spiritual, and physical energies to be more effective through each phase of resting and helps keep you active mentally and spiritually. A side benefit of Lavender is that it can release tension in the neck and shoulders. Find it in our "Peaceful Sleep" blend.

Lemon Balm facilitates deep natural relaxation. It eases the velocity of the mind, helping you slip into an alpha state more easily. Lemon Balm also moves anxiety out so revelation can surface. It is great for children unable to relax or slow down. It calms fears and helps regulate the sleep cycle. Lemon Balm flower essence is a restorer after stress from modern civilization and from being around too many people or stretched too thin. It is for those who struggle with anxiety over something obvious or anxiety over something lurking in the background of the mind. Either way, Lemon Balm helps release peace of mind, usually through dreams. Find it in our "Peaceful Sleep," "Stress Less," "Peace," and "Dream Drops" blends.

Lettuce is a great calmer and helps you communicate clearly and focus. It soothes the central nervous system and eases external stresses. Lettuce also helps unwind kids who are overtired, hyperactive, or too wound up to play constructively. Find it in our "Smoke-Free" and "Peaceful Sleep" blends.

Lilac helps those who won't let others help them. They can't delegate work. "If you want it done right, you have to do it yourself." These people carry a tremendous load and often have back problems. Lilac is often used in conjunction with chiropractic care to help an adjustment last longer. Find it in our "Align" blend.

Lovage helps make continual progress in a positive direction. It's all about growth, less talk, and more action. Lovage helps you move forward despite fear when called out of your comfort zone. Use Lovage when there is uncertainty about the direction you should take because Lovage will bring a resonance of strength, joy, and confidence. Find it in our "M&M" blend.

Maltese Cross has large flower heads made up of loads of little red crosses. The signature of this plant denotes that it's applicable when you need some disaster relief or the ability to remember to stand in faith for what is rightfully yours in life. Maltese Cross flower essence renews our confidence that the events in life that are designed to shatter us are actually what can catapult us forward, set us free, and bring us back stronger. Find it in our "Crisis Care" blend.

Malva aids in stopping the cycles of rejection. For many of us, life is always about our perception and not what is necessarily reality. An initial trauma of rejection can sensitize a person to further perceived slights any time people fall short of what is expected in the relationship. This can cause distancing and the mentality of "I'll leave so you can't hurt me." It can also cause hostility, which prompts those they are in relationship with to also become defensive and withdraw. The cycle completes with the person feeling justified in their initial perception. Malva helps to desensitize, soothe, and unravel the reinforced patterns. Stopping the rejection cycle is the only way to obtain what's needed through relationships. Malva prompts the bravery needed to stay and experience the reality that's beyond the initial perception and melt away the paranoia and unloved feelings. Find it in our "Heart Healer" blend.

Marie Pavie Rose goes to those places that are very difficult to access and helps parts of the soul in deep bondage to surface and heal. It instills a sense of peace amid the sometimes tumultuous emotional processing of old trauma. It enables you to hear your soul parts and fragments so that they heal. For SRA survivors, it breaks down energetic blocks and other high-tech operations so that alters can't communicate with each other or with the core personality. It facilitates more restful nights for those who tend to have spiritual battles when they need to be sleeping. Find it in our "Fragment Finder" blend.

Missouri Primrose reaches back to our childhood, helping us to reframe some our circumstances. Many of us were told we would never amount to anything or that we were limited in some way. Others may have grown up with an overall lack of love, abuse, strict religious teachings, or other ways of ensuring we would have a battle over our worth. This sets us up to feel undeserving anytime blessings come our way. Beliefs that something bad will happen because things are too good come from this place, but Missouri Primrose is a master at reshaping all the childhood trauma, reinstating our worthiness, and helping us learn to receive and to self-nurture. Find it in our "Confidence," "Prosper," and "Floral Defense" blends.

Milk Thistle helps you forgive and let go of anger, especially in cases of long-standing family problems. It is effective whether or not you're in touch with your feelings. This essence brings on the dreams and offers a cathartic release. The herb Milk Thistle is used for liver toxicity and poisoning. Similarly, the essence works to cleanse the negative emotions that gravitate to the liver. Find it in our "Anger Management" and "Dream Drops" blends.

Moonbeam Coreopsis is an excellent essence to use during recuperation, whether post-operative, emotional, physical, mental, or spiritual. It facilitates heart rebuilding and depth of the healing process that goes beyond the obvious. Many times, we have physical symptoms that are related to much deeper heart issues. This essence energetically wraps around you and gives you a reassuring hug, helping you receive healing on a deeper level. Find it in our "Aftershock," "Floral Defense," and "Recovery" blends.

Moonshine Yarrow helps keep you immune to other people's anger and negativity. Sometimes when we're angry, we're simply mirroring what's going on around us and making other people's dissatisfaction our own. Find it in our "Anger Management," "Floral Defense," and "Yarrow Shield" blends.

Mullein amplifies your ability to connect with the still small voice, especially in areas of right and wrong and fulfilling your purpose. Decision-making becomes clearer, and your ability to stand strong and stick to your guns is enhanced. Mullein allows a calm certainty and sense of protection as you walk your unique path. For anyone who is indecisive or who has difficulty recognizing the voice of God, Mullein has a way of making blacks blacker and whites whiter. The gray scale goes away, and you can move into action with confidence. Find it in our "Open Ears" blend.

Nasturtium rebalances people who have been deep into intellectual pursuits to the point of exhaustion and feeling disconnected from the world around them. Nasturtium is a great way to wrap up a school year or handle burnout at an overly intellectual job. Nasturtium sometimes can help with obsessive-compulsive disorder (OCD), chronic-fatigue syndrome, and metabolic dysfunction. Find it in our "Ignite" blend.

Nettle takes the sting out of past trauma and helps you identify toxic circumstances in your life. It helps where we have become overly sensitive due to old hurts and get angry, feel tormented, and subsequently disconnect from others. It's especially indicated for those who came from broken homes, abusive situations, or other disturbances to the family unit. If you have present emotions that seem unreasonable given your current situation, trouble maintaining healthy relationships, or generally feel misunderstood, Nettle can help release the pain that's locked in as well as help you establish proper social boundaries.

Nicotiana Yes, it's made from the tobacco flower. Nicotiana flower essence has a long track record of working with addictions, predominately to cigarettes. It helps by strengthening an addictive personality for those who need a substance to cope and making it okay to feel the feelings. Being tough and cool is overrated. So is being the loner. Nicotiana is connecting and grounding, softening, and even a peace maker as Native Americans know. Find it in our "Smoke-Free" blend.

Onion flower essence is great for the grieving process. Onion will release crying if you need to cry and stop you up if you can't quit or if you're holding on to excessive pain and need to move on. It's great because you don't have to try and figure out whether you're reacting appropriately or not; it will balance you. It's very important to grieve fully and completely, but you don't want to cry forever. Onion will help you do what is right for you. Onion is your fastest route through the grieving process. It helps you access your emotions, express them completely, and then move on. It works equally well on present situations and on past bottled-up grief. Find it in our "Good Grief" blend.

Orange Mum fosters helpful energy throughout the day, helps the soul/spirit balance, and works for Body Coaching similarly to our regular Chrysanthemum. Orange Mum in particular seems a bit more active on the physical aspect of the spirit/soul/body combo. It seems to be a regulator of different functions that are either cyclical or rhythmic, such as breathing and women's periods, or fluid-related, like mucus production or hydration. Find it in our "Aunt Flo's Secret Weapon" blend.

Oregon Grape heals patterns of conditioning that are instilled in us, such as conditioning that tells us we aren't safe in relationships and can't let our guard down. Oregon Grape helps you see the good intentions of others and disrupts paranoid thought processes, allowing trust and love to flourish. Find it in our "Heart Healer" blend.

Parrot Tulip flower essence brings about an upbeat positive mood, brimming with get-it-done energy. It helps you find humor and optimism everywhere and enhances social situations. If you're an introvert that has to be around a bunch of people, this will help you act as an extrovert temporarily. If you have to navigate difficult personalities, Parrot Tulip will help you maintain a positive attitude and shrug off the naysayers. The name does have bearing. Some of our testers found that when tossed into difficult situations, they were quickly able to recall and repeat Bible verses, affirmations, and mantras to better face the issues. Find it in our "Joy" blend.

Pear promotes an internal peace, so your inner warrior can rise up and confidently confront your issues head on. Pear also works within relationships to bring resolution. Find it in our "Crisis Care" blend.

Pink Yarrow aids in discerning and separating your own emotions from what you are picking up from others. This helps you set healthy boundaries while remaining compassionate. Find it in our "Yarrow Shield" blend.

Plantain helps release bitterness and resentment. It dissolves negative and repetitive thought patterns that keep you stuck in old cycles. It changes biting words into a more positive means of communication and heals the wounds that have been inflicted by others. This essence helps you get along with others. Find it in our "Peace," "Aunt Flo's Secret Weapon," and "Anger Management" blends.

Plumbago helps people pleasers who often operate under obligation. Those who need Plumbago easily accept shame, blame, and guilt and deal with a level of unworthiness that can shut out blessings. If we want to succeed in life and forge ahead, we need to be able to move past our failures and disappointments. Plumbago helps us to let events take their course and to keep moving forward despite our mistakes. It also helps us when we've lost trust in our own judgement or intuition. Plumbago also helps us restore a sense of autonomy, confidence, and deservedness while maintaining empathy and sensitivity to others' needs. Find it in our "Peak Performance" blend.

Potato helps you take your deep spiritual experiences and bring them into reality and practice. This is a lovely essence to help your spiritual growth continue at a steady rate. Potato counteracts spaciness, daydreaming, escapism, and trouble with seeing the big picture. Potato is grounding, helping you make sense of new or abstract concepts so you can integrate the information into your everyday life. With Potato, the phrase "so heavenly-minded you're no earthly good" applies. The truth is being heavenly-minded makes you a lot of earthly good, but only if you can bring it down to earth in a practical manner. Potato helps you hold on to those insights and act accordingly. Find it in our "Dream Drops" and "Focus" blends.

Prickly Pear flower essence helps lessen emotional reactions to change. It brings an ease so that instead of trying to control all outcomes, we can relax and realize that our best path through is surrender. It helps us focus on the resources at our disposal instead of what we don't have. For that reason, it's perfect for people who tend to overbuy, overeat, or otherwise excessively resource themselves in times of uncertainty or confusion.

Purple Archangel is all about putting matters in order. It clarifies the complex; aids in understanding and decisive action; and simplifies and grounds those who are stuck in chaos. Benefits those dealing with creative blocks, those who are trying to become organized, or those who feel worn out by work or excess activity. For those going in a hundred directions at once who feel the need to decipher what is worthwhile and what is not. Find it in our "M&M" blend.

Queen Anne's Lace is beneficial for anyone wanting to amplify or activate a seer ability. For those who already have a strong gift in this area, Queen Anne's is grounding and balancing between realms. It also enhances discernment and brings balance between overly mystical and rational thinking. Queen Anne's Lace has been reported to clear up physical vision problems as well when the cause is psychosomatic. Find it in our "Vision Quest" blend.

Red Chestnut is indicated whenever you become overly concerned for another person. This usually happens in a parent-child relationship but can occur when you have repetitive or obsessive thoughts and worry about another's well-being. Those that need Red Chestnut often have a hard time with trust in a higher power because the world is a scary place to them. They imagine the worst rather than hoping for the best. Red Chestnut can shift your perspective over time to replace worry with faith.

Red Clover helps you stay calm and think clearly in the midst of pandemonium. Other people's negative energy has a tendency to capture us as well. Think of Red Clover as an inoculation against mob mentality.

Rose Campion is an interesting essence to accompany healing work within the bloodline. It seems to enlighten us regarding our choices as to what we want to receive from our lineage. It helps heal woundings that cycle through the generations. Rose Campion opens pathways between generations via love and forgiveness. For best results, pray, dream, envision, and travel through your bloodline for revelation as to what's there. Through these passageways, we can receive healing as well as our spiritual inheritance.

Rosemary aids you when traumatizing situations have caused a disconnect from the physical realm. For those who don't feel entirely present or in tune with their bodies, Rosemary can bring about a greater healing and a sense of safety for the soul and spirit to inhabit its earthly temple. Forgetfulness, spending a lot of time out-of-body, and hypoglycemic tendencies may be indicators of old trauma that has convinced you that it's not safe to be in the here and now. Rosemary is known as the "herb of remembrance," which reminds you that you are a spirit and soul that has a physical body. I can't not let the re-member pun go by, either, as it helps you reacquaint with every member of your body. Rosemary has a social aspect as well, helping you to reintegrate into your place as a member of a society, network, or community. Find it in our "Healthy Intimacy" blend.

Rue helps us identify deceptive and abusive behavior masquerading as good intentions. It replaces blind faith with true discernment involving those who are impacting our lives or well-being. Rue helps us shake off gaslighting, brainwashing, and other mind games and change the roles we play in the wake of narcissists, those in positions of authority, and charismatic personalities with hidden motives. With Rue, we can more easily see where our boundaries have been lax. Rue's botanical name is *Ruta*, which comes from the Greek word *reuo* and means "to set free." Rue helps us see the truth about our relationships and leaders, and the truth sets us free. Find it in our "Powerhouse" blend.

Russian Sage moves us into a spiritual maturity by helping transition us out of a state of confusion, desolation, and barrenness. It opens up the respiratory system and sets our hearts aflame with love. It starts the movement and diffusion of our affections, gratitude, and joy upward and set on things above, not to be diverted or distracted by the winds of adversity. To be in tune with the Russian Sage frequency is to live from a place of overflow, abundance, and lightness. Issues of unworthiness quietly move out, as easy as exhaling. Find it in our "Joy" and "Prosper" blends.

Self-Heal strengthens your resolve and puts you in charge of your recovery process with a newfound faith for healing. It is a very beneficial remedy for those who face physical, mental, or spiritual healing challenges or anyone who is trying to take better care of themselves. In addition to intuitively tuning you in to what you personally need for healing, never mind the gurus, it helps you take charge and do what you know you need to do to be well and do those things consistently. Sometimes the recovery process is hard. Self-Heal is your personal motivator and cheerleader, instilling in you the will to keep moving forward. Find it in our "Menoblend," "Aftershock," "Align," "Aunt Flo's Secret Weapon," and "Recovery" blends.

Shasta Daisy helps you see how everything fits together in the big picture. It helps you pull pieces of disconnected information, ideas, and concepts together into a cohesive whole. This essence is excellent for writers, researchers, and teachers who need to produce comprehensive, understandable presentations. It's also perfect for multi-taskers and anyone who has to keep track of lots of projects or information. Shasta Daisy assists with compartmentalized emotions and thoughts, helping you reintegrate and become whole rather than shutting down or sectioning off feelings that you can't deal with. When you see the big picture, this can reduce anxiety. Shasta Daisy has been used to prevent panic attacks. Shasta can also restore wholeness in relationships by allowing you to see the big picture there, too, rather than focusing on winning arguments. Find it in our "M&M" and "Vision Quest" blends.

Shooting Stars help those who feel very different from those around them, as in profound alienation or other worldly. They haven't quite mentally or emotionally connected with the earthly realm. Many have had difficult or traumatizing births or womb trauma. They often face a constant though not always obvious battle to fulfill their destiny or purpose, especially early in life. This tends to show up as childhood health issues, and the disconnect between them and others or between them and the divine as well as a disconnect from their true identity and mission to earth. For a Shooting Star personality to step into their purpose, they have to initially battle through a fog of having a strong sense of purpose though not knowing what exactly it is, then potentially the fear of ostracism, ridicule, or even martyrdom. Shooting Star will help you recognize why you are here and help you stand in your identity in the face of opposition as well as feel more connected to the earthly realm and those you share it with. Find it in our "Bravely You" blend.

Skullcap helps those who are self-critical or neglect themselves. It's ideal for parts work, easing into those areas where you've not been able to fully accept yourself, usually due to early trauma. It reinstates sensitivity where there was numbness and allows self-forgiveness and self-nurturing to happen. We're also seeing possibilities of helping with parts that seem absent. Skullcap has a history of helping people overcome addictions, allowing us to find healthier ways of coping, and reducing the emotionally driven cravings and withdrawal symptoms. Skullcap is in our "Fragment Finder" blend.

Snapdragon helps release tension in the jaw area from withholding words and for those with less self-control when it comes to letting abusive words fly. Sarcasm, criticism, teeth grinding, TMJ, and the need to eat hard, crunchy, or chewy foods can indicate a need for Snapdragon essence. Find it in our "Anger Management" blend.

Solomon's Seal helps you relinquish control and attachment to outcomes so you can go with the flow. It helps you move through disappointment and frustration quickly so you can refocus and adjust how you do things. It helps you learn from mistakes, adapt to unforeseen circumstances, and work effectively with circumstances outside your control. Find it in our "Tomorrow" blend.

Sow Thistle helps you deal effectively with inappropriate behavior, whether by you or another person. It helps you stand up to bullies and is helpful in reconciling issues in group situations. Think of Sow Thistle as anti-domineering. Whether it's obnoxious, pushy behavior or a more subtle controlling relationship using manipulation or smothering, Sow Thistle brings the issues into clear focus, helping you make healthy changes. Find it in our "Anger Management" and "Floral Defense" blends.

Speedwell helps people who are moving too fast or having trouble living in the present. It instigates stillness and focus. Speedwell increases spiritual insight and awareness and helps you go at the "right speed." It brings a sense of calm in the midst of chaos and allows you to rest. Speedwell teaches that you can cover a lot of ground by consistently focusing on small tasks without rushing. It also allows you to see ahead and maintain objectivity regarding the vision. Many times, when we receive revelation from the spiritual realm, we immediately try to make sense of it through leaning on our own understanding. Our grids for understanding come from past experience, what we've been taught, religious doctrines, and emotional or cultural mindsets. These can color the vision so that it loses its true meaning in the translation. Speedwell keeps you grounded and better able to see it for what it is. Find it in our "Stress Less" and "Vision Quest" blends.

Star of Bethlehem is the classic trauma essence. Whether old trauma or new, it helps you find reassurance and rapidly neutralizes trauma. Practically all of us experience shocking events in our lives. Star of Bethlehem reverses the shutting down effects of trauma and helps the user regain the ability to cope with circumstances with mental clarity and inner strength. Find it in our "Aftershock," "Crisis Care," "Floral Defense," and "Good Grief" blends.

Star Thistle aids in feeling and focusing on abundance rather than lack. Those who have a tendency to tighten up and be fearful during financial stress, Great Depression survivors, hoarders, or anyone who feels there is not enough to go around will benefit from Star Thistle. Find it in our "Prosper" blend.

St. John's Wort has to do with light in every sense. We use this on people who are sensitive to light, who are afraid of the dark, and who are deprived of light, such as for S.A.D. or graveyard workers. Saint John's not only deals with external physical light but brings light inward, illuminating your soul. The Greek name for this plant is *Hypericum* (which is also its Latin botanical name) and means "over a spirit." It has a very long history of offering spiritual protection, protection against nightmares, and helping people face darkness. I believe this to be more of a solidifying of courage and authority rather than a mere superstition. The common name came about because its peak harvest time happens on St. John's Day. Whether you're harvesting for a flower essence or as an herb, the flowering tops are used. When the flower heads are picked, the plant oozes a bright red sap, depicting the beheading of John the Baptist. This signature refers to helping one keep their head or spiritual authority at those times when negative spiritual influences seek to cut us off.

Sunflower addresses father wounds and heals distortions in authority relationships. When we grow up with a conflicted relationship or lack of relationship to our fathers, this affects our self-esteem. We also tend to project the natural relationship we had with our fathers onto how we see God. None of us had perfect fathers in the natural; our issues may cause a block in our ability to receive from the Father, who is perfect. Insecurity might also be an issue so that the person continually tries to convince others of their value. Sunflower corrects both insecurity and pride, bringing the person into balance in the grand scheme of things. Find it in our "Confidence," "Peak Performance," and "Open Ears" blends.

Sweet Cherry is a broad-spectrum negative emotions essence, dissolving fear, anger, and frustration. It strengthens you to see goodness and softens your heart toward others. It takes down walls of self-protection that keep you from relating properly with others. Find it in our "Peace" and "Anger Management" blends.

Sweet Chestnut is helpful during those dark nights of the soul when feelings of intense despair and of being utterly alone are pervasive. Use this essence when you have no sense of understanding from others and no sense of higher guidance. If you feel there is no way out, no hope, and you are at a breaking point, Sweet Chestnut helps break down old patterns and belief systems, restores faith, and helps you realize that a new path and change is possible.

Sweet Pea helps people who are unable to form social bonds or figure out where they fit in. Used by frequent travelers who are homesick and by those who hop from one thing to another without becoming truly involved, Sweet Pea offers a sense of roots and connectedness. Sweet Pea is also a great aid for kids and pets that have just undergone a move and need to settle in and make new friends. Find it in our "Bravely You" blend.

Sweet William aids in stopping cycles of negative thoughts regarding past woundings and dwelling on or stirring up pain. We can build up false expectations either by being sure we will always be hurt or by also perceiving every little misstep from another as an intentional stab. It sets the stage for more realistic expectations in future relationships. Find it in our "Heart Healer" blend.

Tansy helps ward off procrastination and indecision. When you experience chaos, confusion, emotional instability, or violence, it's normal to back away and withdraw. On the surface, this looks like apathy and laziness, but it may be symptomatic of a deeper issue, perhaps one ingrained from childhood. Tansy addresses the functional side of the core personality after fragmentation and helps you feel empowered and purposeful with fresh energy and an attitude conducive to success. It helps users take decisive action and helps them get back in the game. Find it in our "M&M" blend.

Teasel is for depleted, emotionally-exhausted people. The key with this remedy is loss of energy through any emotional condition, strained relationship, or long term illness. Another plus of Teasel is that it gives you the good sense to live and work in the livelihood Creator calls you to. When you're working in the wrong field, your energy isn't being restored. Teasel helps you find the place that resonates with your spirit. When taking Teasel, a person may sometimes become solitary or withdrawn. This is all part of the process. It's a place of restoration and reflection on how to change situations, relationships, and your behavior to a more sustainable lifestyle. Use Teasel when you have lost energy or deal with aches and pains. There is also a lot of documented use of Teasel flower essence as a complementary therapy for Lyme disease. Teasel helps children learn to regulate their energy and helps those that are hyper-active and then drop when exhausted. It helps stabilize them so that they find a more moderate pace for playing and resting. Find it in our "Recovery" blend.

Thimbleberry supports an easy-going, look-on-the-bright-side mentality and gives you the ability to be unfazed by difficult circumstances. You will have the attitude of "Que sera sera!" Thimbleberry supports a detachment to imagined outcomes with the philosophy that everything ultimately works out for the best. Increased awareness of angelic activity adds to the confidence that the details are being taken care of. It lets you flow through life with positivity, joy, and gratitude. Find it in our "Joy" blend.

Tiger Lily helps balance mood swings and hot flashes. It brings stability and harmony by allowing the user to let go of hostility and aggressive tendencies. It has a long history of balancing hormonal tension. Find it in our "Menoblend" and "Aunt Flo's Secret Weapon" blends.

Tithonia gives you the confidence to creatively do your own thing. No backing down from self-doubt or sabotaging yourself. Tithonia gives us the courage to go for it—in a big way. It's perfect for those who are exploring new things and developing new skills. Find it in our "Ignite" blend.

Trumpet Vine assists in speaking with confidence and fluidity, broadcasting your personality through a megaphone, and bantering dynamically and synergistically with others. Words can be compared to seeds. Trumpet Vine creates big pods that snap open on a precise timetable. It is also helpful for those trying to communicate through art or other non-verbal means and for those trying to teach or explain a difficult concept. It helps with intimidation and shyness, and it may help with speech impediments or when trying to learn a new language. Find it in our "Confidence" blend.

Verbena ameliorates stiff, rigid conceptual thinking and the inability to find tenderness with loved ones. It helps release hostility, judgments, and hardened attitudes. Those who lead and teach by shaming or displaying rigid, overbearing behavior and high expectations can release their inner taskmaster and find less abrasive methods of communication for more playful, sincere life and creativity.

Violet strengthens the introverts, the shy ones, the so-called shrinking violets. Introverts have to maintain a tension between sharing one's self and one's gift to the world with the downtime and solitude needed to develop those things in private. I spoke in the beginning of this book of the flower as the reproductive apparatus of a plant. But violets are the exception—sort of. They put out the showy ta-da! flower that we all love, but they have few, if any, seeds. The real reproduction goes on beneath the leaf canopy with unseen and petalless flowers full of seeds. This is reflective of the way violet personalities function best. The outward flower is for the rest of us to love and delight in yet protects the most important development until ready to be unleashed. For this reason, violet is great not only for the shy but for the artists, writers, and others who desire privacy during creation yet who also need to feel safe enough to share their work.

Wild Aztec Tobacco deals with fears regarding one's relationship with God. It helps facilitate the transition from structured religion to authentic spirituality and all of the fear that holds you back from that freedom by bringing up the event that initially triggered the fear so that you can take it before God and consciously deal with it. This essence also helps gifted children so they don't suppress their spiritual side when they receive negative feedback from others. Find it in our "Dream Drops" blend.

Wild Rose flower essence assists where there has been a shut down and the person is resigned to their current situation, unable to see any way out. There is no fight in them, only acceptance of their fate as inevitable. Wild Rose brings life back in with a new-found inner freedom to live life to its fullness even though it is filled with trials. Find it in our "Tomorrow" and "Ignite" blends.

Wisteria is an appetite stimulant that also reveals how and why we should set better boundaries. It helps us discern our blind spots and gives us greater insight into our current troublesome situations. Wisteria also opens our emotions while not allowing them to cloud our judgement. The result is a stronger stance against co-dependency, denial, and false responsibility.

White Chestnut helps users get off the mental merry-go-round when they have a to-do list swimming in their heads at all times and constant mind chatter adding to stress, White Chestnut calms and clears the thinking. It's appropriate for those with OCD and for those with busy minds. White Chestnut can tame the worries, give you confidence to solve daily problems, and help you realize that challenges are opportunities to grow. White Chestnut is a remedy for insomnia, too, if your thought life keeps you up at night. Find it in our "Peaceful Sleep," "Focus," and "Stress Less" blends.

Wormwood helps us transition from the dream state to waking and allows for better dream recall. Wormwood is also useful for processing unresolved issues and helps with letting go of the past. Find it in our "Dream Drops" blend.

Xhosa, also known as African Dream Root, means "white ways/white paths" and is a plant native to the Eastern Cape of South Africa, where it is regarded by the Xhosa people as sacred. Its root is traditionally used to induce vivid (and according to the Xhosa, prophetic) dreams. This is the flower essence, so no alkaloids are present in this form. Find it in our "Dream Drops" blend.

Yarrow helps sensitive people be less affected by other's moods and less-than- harmonious environments. It sets boundaries for those who are empathetic and those in healing/care-giving arenas where they pick up other people's issues or land issues and are deeply affected by them. I believe that what's diagnosed as mental or social disorders might sometimes actually be sensitivity to environmental and energetic conditions. In these cases, Yarrow can be beneficial. It may also strengthen those who have other conditions relating to their environment, such as multiple chemical sensitivities and allergies. Find it in our "Yarrow Shield" blend.

Yellow Monkey Flower is a classic remedy for fears, phobias, and anxiety. If you can specifically name your fear as opposed to dealing with mysterious panic attacks with no explanation, then Yellow Monkey Flower will help you face it with joy and humor. It calms the fight-or-flight response and releases us into greater levels of joy and curiosity. Yellow Monkey Flower tends to be most appropriate for sensitive, introverted individuals. Find it in our "Stay Calm," "Craving Control," and "Prosper" blends.

Zinnia helps you lighten up and laugh more. Laughter, as we all know, is the best medicine. For anyone who takes him or herself too seriously or who has lost their sense of playfulness or adventure, zinnia restores these. It is a very good essence for the elderly, the workaholic, the bored, those who don't relate well to children, or anyone with depression. Encouraging spontaneity and silliness, Zinnia is just plain fun. Bridging the gap between the responsible adult and the inner child is what Zinnia does best. Find it in our "Joy" blend.

All essences can be found at www.freedom-flowers.com. Custom blends are available, or you can do a DIY option of putting any seven flowers that you like into one bottle on this page. http://bit.ly/DIYcombo

Flower essence practitioner training is also available if you'd like to help others.

BOUQUET BLENDS

These are the most economical and convenient way to get started with flower essences. They combine several flowers in one bottle for specific and common issues. They are available at http://bit.ly/bouquetblends

Aftershock is the essence for repairing and restoring after any kind of deeply emotional shock, old or new. Recommended for, but not limited to, war vets, victims of abuse, accidents, or sexual crimes.

Align helps with emotions that tend to manifest in back, neck, and shoulder pain or misalignment. Helps to maximize the benefits from chiropractic, massage, or other healing modalities.

Anger Management flower essence blend helps get rid of rage, repressed anger, resentment, and irritation.

Aunt Flo's Secret Weapon helps reduce moodiness, irritability, tearfulness, and cramping associated with your monthly cycle.

Bravely You helps you stand in your individual identity and be more comfortable being yourself, especially if you feel as if you've always had trouble fitting in.

Confidence is for self-assurance, self-respect, recognition of your own worth, and for shyness and difficulty expressing yourself.

Craving Control helps foster a healthy mindset and proper motivation and addresses the emotional aspects of stress eating, addiction, and self-medicating. Not only is it helpful with eating disorders but it is ideal for anyone who wants to have a healthier relationship with food.

Crisis Care can help a person stay calm and think clearly to deal with the crisis at hand. Helpful for accidents, tragedies, crimes, and traumatizing situations.

Dream Drops helps those who, for whatever reason, have trouble recalling dreams. Dreams can be a critical to healing, getting life direction, and stepping into your destiny. This is a great essence for those who have had some kind of repression due to fear of nightmares or fear of deception.

Floral Defense is designed to repair past damage from abuse and to guard the heart from the effects of further abuse. It gradually restores self-worth and identity while energetically wrapping around you like a warm blanket of love.

Focus may help mental clarity, memory, concentration, attention issues, hyperactivity, and brain imbalance. Ideal for those whose lifestyle demands sustained mental focus, such as students, writers, office workers, and teachers; those who experience the post-lunch slump, and as a complementary therapy for those with learning disorders or mental confusion.

Fragment Finder is used to bring about a resolution to buried emotional wounds that have caused the formation of soul splits or fragments and alters by bringing these matters to light. Its action varies from "flushing out the bushes" and bringing up a split in your soul that needs to be addressed to spontaneous integration and healing.

Good Grief is a blend of very comforting essences to release you from the effects of shock. Use in the event of a death or breakup or when dealing with a loss.

Healthy Intimacy addresses a range of sexual and relational issues due to past trauma, generational trauma, and conditioned beliefs concerning sex and love.

Heart Healer eases the pain of heartbreak, abandonment, rejection, and co-dependency.

Ignite flower essence lights up your passion, your creativity, your vision, and your zest for life. Combining hot colored, super energy flowers with those that produce peppery hot flavors, this blend dislodges negative stagnant ruts we sometimes fall into.

Joy flower essence blend is for bubbling up joy and laughter despite circumstances. This flower remedy helps you pull out of situational depression and gloomy moods.

M&M (Motivation and Manifestation) combats procrastination, indecision, and feelings of being stuck. It aids in multi-tasking, not losing sight of the forest for the trees, and setting plans of action. It builds confidence in talents and decision-making and gives you the confidence to forge ahead.

Menoblend helps with emotional and physical symptoms of menopause or a recent hysterectomy.

Open Ears deals with common blocks to spiritual hearing and amplifies your ability to tune into divine guidance and make decisions.

Peace eases stress, anxiety, frustration, and anger. Facilitates getting along with others. It's a great essence blend for the majority of us that have to interact with other people that aren't our favorites.

Peaceful Sleep assists those with busy minds. It eases cyclical thought patterns, worry, and the need to understand everything right now.

Peak Performance clears out the programming from close relationships when you may have felt love was contingent on you acting a certain way. When you break free of these constructs, you are free to follow your original design and be the amazing person that you were created to be.

Powerhouse helps with personal empowerment, free thinking, and healing victimization/victim mentality. For those who look to other people or systems to support or balance them as well as those who simply want to strengthen their own sense of freedom, accomplishment, and autonomy.

Prosper addresses poverty mentality, scarcity, and lack. It is about money but goes so much deeper than that. Prosper helps you tap into abundance in all areas of your life by working on your heart issues around your own worth and what you really think about money.

Recovery is support and strengthening during illness. Encourages a positive overcomer attitude, alleviates health-related fears, and helps you get in touch with what your body, mind, and spirit need for total healing.

Smoke-Free provides strength, de-stressing, and motivation while addressing addictive tendencies for those quitting smoking or vaping.

Stay Calm supports those prone to anxiety. It calms nerves, stops obsessive thinking patterns, instills courage, and relaxes the overactive mind.

Stress Less helps those who have a hard time relaxing and helps find ways to build a healthier lifestyle that's more conducive to their own well-being.

Vision Quest helps with spiritual vision, finding life's purpose, and breakthrough.

Yarrow Shield is beneficial for those who are sensitive to environments and other people's moods and energies. Establishes safe boundaries and is protective against intentional attack or passive absorption.

THANK YOU!

A big thanks for reading this book and seeing it through to the end. I'd like to ask a small favor. Could you please take a minute or two and leave a review on Amazon?

Your feedback will help me continue to write books that help you get results. If you found the information valuable, please let me know.

Seneca

Endnotes

1 James Strong, Strong's Exhaustive Concordance of the Bible, "rachaph, (H7363)," (Nashville: Abingdon Press, 1890).

2 James Strong, Strong's Exhaustive Concordance of the Bible, "tohuw, (H8414)," (Nashville: Abingdon Press, 1890).

3 L. Montagnier, J. Aïssa, S. Ferris, J. L. Montagnier, and C. Lavallée, "Electromagnetic signals are produced by aqueous nanostructure derived from bacterial DNA sequences," Interdiscip Sci Compu Life Sci no. 1, 2009, 80–91.

4 Thomas Quackenbush, Relearning to See: Improve Your Eyesight Naturally! (Berkley, CA: North Atlantic Books, 2000).

5 Bruce Lipton, "The Jump From Cell Culture to Consciousness," Integrative Medicine: A Clinician's Journal," 2017 Dec; 16(6): 44–50, https://www.ncbi.nlm.nih.gov/pmc/articles/PMC6438088/.

6 Bessel A. van der Kolk, The Body Keeps the Score: Brain, Mind, and Body in the Healing of Trauma, (New York: Viking, 2014).

7 Carsten Spitzer, Stefanie Wegert, Jürgen Wollenhaupt, Katja Wingenfeld, Sven Barnow, Hans Joergen Grabe, "Gender-specific association between childhood trauma and rheumatoid arthritis: A case–control study," Journal of Psychosomatic Research, April 2013.

8 Paul Pearsall, The Heart's Code: Tapping the Wisdom and Power of Our Heart Energy, (New York: Harmony, 1999)

9 V. E. Lloyd, "The Jarisch-Herxheimer Reaction," The British Journal of Venereal Diseases, vol. 21,1 (1945): 42-4. doi:10.1136/sti.21.1.42.

10 Jacob Bohme, The Signature of All Things: De Signatura Rerum, (Germany, 1621).

ABOUT THE AUTHOR

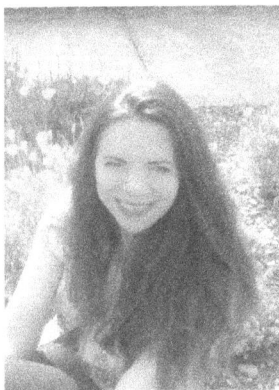

Seneca Schurbon

Seneca started making and selling flower essences at the ripe old age of five. Her company Freedom Flowers, based in the Idaho wilderness, is the perfect marriage of the natural and spiritual for emotional healing. She actively works to take back the things of God that have been ceded over to the enemy, by looking for Gods original purpose for his creation. Seneca also enjoys research rabbit trails, exploring ideas, and dragging others along for the ride.

FB: www.facebook.com/freedomfloweressence
Instagram: @FreedomFlowerEssence
Website: www.Freedom-Flowers.com

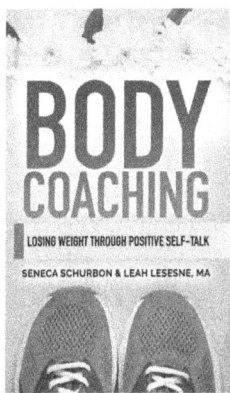

Body Coaching: Losing Weight Through Positive Self-talk

"Body, we need to talk..."

What we say to ourselves and about ourselves matters. Body coaching is a 30-day program of positive self-talk. Taking authority in our spirits over our bodies and giving ourselves the pep talks we've desperately needed.

It's not about will powering your way through another diet or exercise program, it's about partnering your body, mind, and spirit together so that you can experience the breakthroughs you've been longing for.

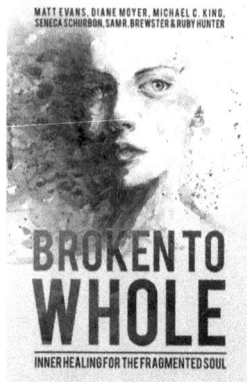

MATT EVANS, DIANE MOYER, MICHAEL C. KING,
SENECA SCHURBON, SAM R. BREWSTER & RUBY HUNTER

BROKEN TO WHOLE

INNER HEALING FOR THE FRAGMENTED SOUL

Broken to Whole: Inner Healing for the Fragmented Soul

Why Aren't You Healed?

Do you ever feel like you continually struggle with certain emotions? Maybe you've tried counseling or various ministries, yet no matter what you do, nothing works.

If traditional prayer and deliverance hasn't cut it, you might be dealing with soul fragments. When we experience a traumatizing event, part of our coping strategy is to wall off a little piece of ourselves in order to contain that emotion. We then go on with life. A fragment is that part of you that's been locked away, inaccessible to healing, until now.

This book is a game-changer in how you'll look at inner healing. We aren't going to beat the drum for repentance and forgiveness although those are beneficial and necessary. Instead, we have made every effort to tell you something you don't know so that you can fill in your missing pieces.

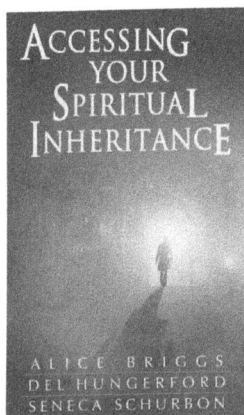

Accessing Your Spiritual Inheritance

It's Your Turn to Go Through the Door

Alice didn't fall down a rabbit hole but she did walk through a mystical doorway in a vision to recover blessings her ancestors failed to claim. When Alice came back and shared her experience, Seneca wasted no time going through her own door. Del's approach differed -- she wound up floating along in her bloodstream!

Through the map we give in our stories, others went through their own doors, leading to better relationships with God, increase in finances, favor, and giftings. Although this book touches on generational curses and how to remove them, we focus on claiming the blessings your family line has lost. However, you'll need to be open to having a vision, and we'll walk you through the step-by-step process of learning to see, so that you, too, can restore your lost generational blessings.

Your hidden inheritance awaits!

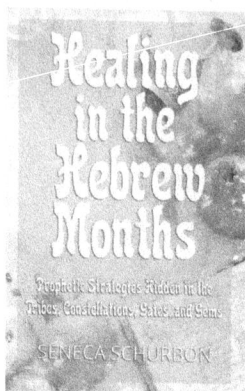

Healing in the Hebrew Months

Get in sync with God's timing! Learn the spiritual rhythms of each season and get new strategy to break free of old and painful cycles.

Have you ever considered there might be a pattern to seemingly random "windows of opportunity"? Or that there are specific times where you can be more easily healed or become free in a certain area? We have been given an actionable template for our lives and spiritual walk. Moreover, this template has confirmed itself for millennia in the stars, tribes, gates of Jerusalem, and the history of each month.

- In each month you'll discover:
- The area of healing most accessible at that time
- The action needed on your part
- Strategic flower essences to use during that month
- God's intention for you in your current situation
- The warfare tactics that are likely to come up
- How to trade the obstacle for opportunity
- The redemptive purpose of the constellations and gemstones

Buy Healing in the Hebrew Months to move towards God's promises for you today!

www.ingramcontent.com/pod-product-compliance
Lightning Source LLC
Chambersburg PA
CBHW050732030426
42336CB00012B/1529